SKINNY

Schedule Me

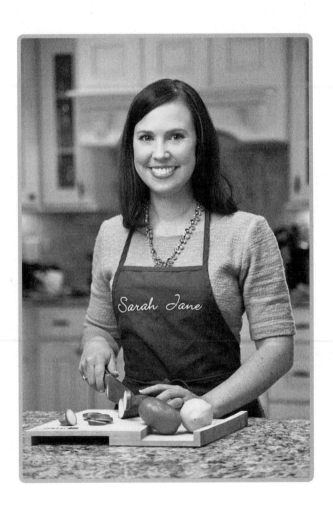

SKINNY

Schedule Me

> **PLAN TO LOSE WEIGHT AND KEEP IT OFF** IN JUST MINUTES A WEEK **30**

SARAH-JANE BEDWELL
RD, LDN

NEW AMERICAN LIBRARY

New American Library
Published by the Penguin Group
Penguin Group (USA) LLC, 375 Hudson Street,
New York, New York 10014

USA | Canada | UK | Ireland | Australia | New Zealand | India | South Africa | China
penguin.com
A Penguin Random House Company

First published by New American Library,
a division of Penguin Group (USA) LLC

First Printing, January 2014

REGISTERED TRADEMARK—MARCA REGISTRADA

LIBRARY OF CONGRESS CATALOGING-IN-PUBLICATION DATA:

Bedwell, Sarah-Jane.
Schedule me skinny: plan to lose weight and keep it off in just
30 minutes a week/Sarah-Jane Bedwell, RD, LDN.
p. cm.
Includes index.
ISBN 978-0-451-46795-9
1. Reducing diets—Recipes. 2. Weight loss. 3. Strategic planning. I. Title.
RM222.2.B425 2014
613.2'5—dc23   2013034983

Printed in the United States of America
1   3   5   7   9   10   8   6   4   2

Set in Warnock Pro
Designed by Susan Hood

CONTENTS

SKINNY

Schedule Me

INTRODUCTION

Women are busier than ever. We have tons of demands on our time and energy—from fast-paced careers to active kids to social commitments. While all of these are the components of a full, rich life, with a schedule this hectic, it can be hard to make time to take care of ourselves. Something has to give to make it all work. And the sacrifice usually comes at a steep price—our health and fitness.

The truth is, though, no matter how much we would like to, we cannot make more time in our day and we still have to keep our commitments. I'm not going to ask you to change your life and totally rearrange your schedule. In this book, I offer you tools and tips to help you incorporate healthy eating and habits into your busy lifestyle without giving up all the fun and excitement of living a full life.

You will have a week's worth of healthy meals planned and prepped in just 30 minutes per week. You will have go-to snack options to energize your afternoon without derailing your diet. You will have strategies for smart choices at any restaurant you select—whether it be Mexican, Asian, or Italian. You will have "Plan B" recipes for nights that don't go as expected that allow you to throw together a healthy dinner in about 30 minutes or less using items from your pantry and freezer. And most important, you will lose up to eight pounds this month alone without deprivation!

The goal of this book is not to starve you to the point of emaciation, but rather to empower you to feel strong, healthy, and in control. You will learn the right balance of healthy, easy meals and on-the-go snacks to help you become a healthier you. Strong really is the new skinny. With this plan, you'll get fit, strong, and lean—revealing a healthy, happy, "skinny" new you!

You see, I wrote this book because I have a busy life myself. For too long, I was at the mercy of my hectic schedule and thought I had no choice but to sacrifice my health. I felt out of control, and I couldn't find the time to create a healthier lifestyle.

It all came to a head at 6:53 p.m. on a Thursday night. I was sitting in the drive-through at Taco Bell wondering what I was doing there. I was spending hours each day studying nutrition and interning under registered dietitians, as well as counseling people on how important it was to put good food in their bodies. So when it came to the food I was putting in my own body, why on earth was I at a drive-through?

My husband and I were newlyweds, and he had just started his first job. I was finishing up my last semester of grad school, driving two hours round-trip to go to classes each day and studying at night. It still amazes me that I also trained for and completed a marathon during that time! I wanted to practice what I preached and prepare healthy meals, but I just couldn't seem to squeeze that into my busy schedule. I was always so tired at the end of the day, and I barely had time to eat, much less cook. Plus, our apartment had such a small kitchen and no dishwasher. The thought of hand-washing all those dishes was too much to bear.

Breakfast was usually just a sugary cereal bar in the car on the way to school. For lunch, I would grab something in the hospital cafeteria where I was interning. Dinner, despite my good intentions, usually ended up being a frozen meal at best or, on the not so good nights, fast food.

The number on the scale was creeping up, and every morning I was waking up feeling sluggish, never with enough energy to make it through the day. I would soon be taking my boards to become a registered dietitian, a licensed expert trained to help others find their way to eating healthfully. But that Thursday night, in line at the drive-through window, I had finally had enough! I knew I couldn't let this continue. Professionally, I wanted to be able to walk the walk and not just talk the talk. And personally, I knew I would feel better, be healthier, and have more energy if I could just make improvements to what I was eating. There had to be a way to make healthy eating work for me.

I turned my car around and drove out of the drive-through line. I went to the grocery store and picked up a rotisserie chicken and a bagged salad for dinner. Hey, it was a start! I made small changes that would lead to big results. I started that weekend by making a grocery list. Within a month, I was planning quick and healthy meals each week. And six months later, I had developed new habits and was fitter and more energetic than ever before.

I discovered the power of planning—the true secret to eating healthy and getting fit when there is no time to spare. I used to think planning would consume more of my precious time, but I found that with just 10 minutes of meal planning, 5 minutes of composing a strategic grocery list, and 15 minutes to prep food at the beginning of each week, I was on the road to a healthy lifestyle in just 30 minutes a week. I quickly realized I didn't have time NOT to take those 30 minutes each week to plan.

I combined my expertise as a registered dietitian and personal experimentation to devise tricks and plans to fit healthier meals into my busy schedule as a consultant dietitian. That prepared me well for the many clients that came into my office expressing the same sentiment: "I really want to lose weight, and I know what I should be doing, but I just don't have the time to do it."

With my realistic approach and easy-to-follow plan, I helped clients lose hundreds of pounds. I showed them how to use a mix-and-match meal pattern so that they could stick with their plan no matter whether they were eating at home, at the ballpark, or at a party. I taught them to devise "Plan B" options for nights when their plans fell through, which helped them feel that they were in control and led them to success in reaching their goals. All the while, they were telling me that they couldn't believe how easy it was. They had all been on diets before, but had never seen the weight come off until now.

Why? Diets have traditionally made it hard to be successful if you have a busy schedule. They usually require extensive meal planning, complicated recipes, and eating five or six times a day. Who has time for that? I know I don't! Today, we women have to live with more expectations than in decades past. Not only are we still serving as the primary homemakers for our families, but now nearly 60% of us work outside the home as well. Add caring for a pet, exercising, travel, and trying to squeeze in time for a social life or romance and there is just no time for counting calories or preparing complex recipes.

REAL-LIFE SUCCESS STORY

When I met Sarah-Jane a few years ago, I was a busy full-time working mother with three teenaged daughters, AND I was experiencing the ups and downs of early menopause. It was a challenging and demanding time for me. With school events, sports practices, housework, and my own job, I felt like I had absolutely no time for myself. Sarah-Jane empowered me. She took the time to get to know me and my daughter

Hilary through weekly visits and the simple use of a food diary. She gave both of us practical steps that were easy and actually worked. I learned that success really is about simple planning—having healthy snacks on hand and keeping a lot of color on your plate. I also learned that it was okay to make my own health a priority. After working with Sarah-Jane, I lost thirty pounds and dropped my cholesterol by fifty [points]. I will use the tools and visuals for the rest of my life. I feel great, and I've learned that small life changes and habits pay off far more than a temporary diet ever could!

—*Jennifer M.*

TIP FROM JENNIFER: Always keep a stash of healthy snacks at work and home. It will make it easier to make healthy choices, and it will prevent you from going too long without eating, which can lead to overeating later.

We've all been tempted by fad diets before. I mean, who doesn't want to believe that you could actually lose twenty pounds in one week? We are bombarded with false promises from such diets. According to them, if we just cut out an entire food group, do a juice cleanse, or simply don't eat for two days each week, the weight will magically fall off. Even though these methods may sound like the easy way up front, anyone who has tried them knows that not only are they torture but they simply do not work.

Let's face it—in our hearts we all know that moderation and balance are the keys to a healthy way of life and weight loss. We know that depriving ourselves now only leads to bingeing later on. If we want to keep the weight off once we lose it, our healthy eating pattern has to become a way of life not just a diet. But it can seem difficult to put moderation and balance into action, especially when you have an unbelievably busy schedule. While it may seem easier to go to the extremes and cut out an entire food group or just skip eating altogether, you can't stick to those methods for the long haul. If you try it, you'll probably end up right back where you started, with extra weight and no solutions. This book will help you find solutions. For the first time, balance and moderation will be easy to understand and even easier to put on your plate. I'll give you the tools you need to succeed, and you will look and feel great because you will know you are losing weight the right way and creating a happy, healthy lifestyle for yourself in the process. I will give you the "skinny" on planning your own way to success! You give me 30 minutes a week, and I will help you lose weight, gain energy, and—most important—develop a healthy lifestyle that lasts.

If, as you read this right now, you find yourself overscheduled and overweight, please know that you are not alone. I've been there and my clients have been there. I want you to know it is not your fault. You've never been given a plan that is realistic for you as a busy, accomplished woman. Never, that is, until now.

 ## Real-life success story

n 2011, I found myself at an extremely low point. I was unhealthy and on the verge of being overweight. I was absolutely miserable. I knew I had to make a change.

I was over thirty-two years old, had spent the last three years in an extremely high-stress job as a nurse practitioner, and had been making very poor dietary choices for the past five years. I finally worked up the nerve to reach out to Sarah-Jane and ask for help. Change is never easy for me. I was worried about feeling deprived, judged, and criticized.

From the day I showed up at Sarah-Jane's door, I never felt any of those things. I learned many things from Sarah-Jane about healthy eating and lifestyle adjustments. I learned that I had to eat something at least every four to five hours, which was difficult for me at work. I actually set an alarm on my phone to remind me. Fruit-and-nut mixes became an easy favorite that I could stick in my pocket. Laughing Cow cheese stuffed into those tiny little peppers was another great snack. Portion control was paramount. I had been pouring myself two or three servings of cereal for breakfast in the morning. That was just the tip of the iceberg! But my favorite tip from Sarah-Jane was finding out that I could drink my favorite caffeinated, high-calorie beverage, Coca-Cola, as long as the serving size was between 100 and 200 calories. I was in heaven. A lifestyle change I could live with. Sign me up! I still use these tips today.

I've lost thirty pounds. My energy level has drastically improved. I actually went to see my doctor the other day and his nurse noticed my weight loss before I even got on the scale. Hearing "You look great, girl!" never, ever gets old. I thought I didn't have the time to make a change and that I was under too much stress to make it work, but I did.

—*Andrea P.*

TIP FROM ANDREA: If you have a busy, stressful schedule like me and want to lose weight and boost your metabolism, remember to eat every four to five hours. I find that setting an alarm on my phone is a great way to remind me to take the time to take care of myself and fuel my body with healthy foods.

Read on. I'll share the plan, tools, and tricks that have worked for me and countless clients despite our busy schedules. You'll see how easy healthy eating can be, even on the busiest of days. Having an eating plan should enable you to succeed, not make you feel like a failure because it is impossible to achieve. My promise to you is that this book will equip you with a realistic approach that enables you to succeed and feel better than you ever have before.

This book will change the way you think about healthy eating. You'll find that following my balanced meal pattern will increase your energy levels, improve your appearance, and allow you to shed one to two pounds of fat each week. You'll lose weight while eating delicious, fresh foods and enjoying a daily treat of your choice, not by depriving yourself. You'll be motivated not just to lose the weight now but to keep it off. That's because this book is the tool you've been searching for to help you find lasting weight loss. It is not a diet; it is a plan for living a full and fit life.

You hold in your hand not only this plan, but also the real-world application in the form of a list of go-to healthy meal and snack options to enjoy whether you have 5 minutes or 50 minutes to spare. No more counting calories. No more hunger pangs. No more guilt. Just results.

THE POWER OF PLANNING

When I started writing this book, one of the things I knew for sure was that I was not going to tell you to count calories, carb grams, or anything else, for that matter. I learned early on in working with clients that if I started talking nutrition by the numbers, their eyes would quickly glaze over.

While it is true that weight loss happens because of a simple equation—calories burned are greater than calories consumed—solving the equation isn't quite so easy. It's not just about counting calories; it's about making calories count by eating the right balance of healthy foods, as each food group plays a specific role in keeping us fit and healthy. Plus, if you focus more on making your calories count rather than trying to count them, the equation usually works itself out (which is a good thing, as math has never been one of my favorite subjects!).

Balance is the key to making your calories count. Every food group has a unique purpose in nourishing our bodies. That's why I tell clients that it's a red flag when a diet or eating plan calls for cutting out an entire food group (like carbs or fat). What I'm presenting to you in this book is not a diet. Instead, it's a simple way of eating real, healthy food despite a busy schedule. Before you know it, eating well will be effortless. It will become your lifestyle and won't require a second thought. The best part is that you will be reaping the benefits. This first month of your new lifestyle, you'll lose up to eight unwanted pounds and feel years younger, thanks to improved energy levels!

I've seen it work for countless busy women, and I know it can work for you too. And unlike those fad diets that ask you to exclude entire food groups or drink your dinner in the form of a weird "chocolate" shake that does NOT taste like its namesake, you'll be eating real, satisfying foods from every delicious food group. This book will prove to you that weight loss does not require deprivation!

The *Schedule Me Skinny* meal pattern provides you with an easy way to achieve this type of balance: fill half your plate with fruits and vegetables, a quarter of your plate with a starch, and a quarter of your plate with protein. You'll use healthy fats and herbs and spices to add flavor to your meals.

Filling half your plate with fruits and veggies provides your body with the essential vitamins and minerals it needs, not only to function optimally but also to keep your metabolism and energy levels going strong. Nutrient-rich produce also is relatively low in calories, yet high in fiber. It takes a long time for the body to digest fiber, so it stays in your stomach longer, keeping you feeling full longer. This means that by filling half your plate with fruits and veggies, you'll need fewer calories to satisfy your hunger, and consuming fewer calories is the key to weight loss. As an added bonus, research shows, people who eat at least 34 grams of fiber per day absorb 6% fewer calories!

The starch on your plate has an important role to play as well. Starchy foods like whole-grain bread, potatoes, or oatmeal provide your body with an easy-to-access energy source to keep your metabolism burning strong. Starches also cause the brain to release a hormone called serotonin, which helps you to feel satisfied after a meal and keeps cravings and mindless munching at bay.

The quarter of your plate that will be filled with protein is key, as protein gives your meal even more staying power. Studies show that getting a quarter of your daily calories from protein helps your body to maintain lean muscle mass, and the more lean muscle mass you have, the better your metabolism is at burning fat. Not only that, but it takes a lot of work for the body to break protein down, so you actually burn double the calories in digesting protein-rich foods that you do in digesting other foods. The body can only use about 15 to 30 grams of protein at a time for burning fat and building lean muscle, making it essential to eat protein with every meal.

Not only does eating healthy fats add flavor, but eating the right types of fat (more on the different types in Chapter 2) can actually help you burn fat. Healthy fats help to keep blood sugar levels steady, which in turn controls hunger. Plus, research shows that healthy fats may promote the activity of the genes in our body that are responsible for burning flab. Healthy fats also promote overall health, including heart health, and the healthier your body is, the better it can function and the more efficient it will be at burning fat. Including some healthy fat in every meal also helps to prevent overeating, as studies show that healthy fats promote satiety.

The secret to making this balanced way of eating work for you is 30 minutes of planning each week. Hands down, among my clients, the ones who have the most success reaching their weight loss or health goals are the ones who follow my advice to set aside one day each week as their meal-planning and grocery-shopping day. For me, this day is Saturday. It's my time to set myself up for a successful week and shop for healthy foods to stock my kitchen. It does take a little time to do, but just by investing 30 minutes once a week on planning, you'll be set for the whole week! Many of my clients tell me they don't have time to plan their meals, but after working with me and seeing both the number on the scale and their stress level drop, they quickly realize they can't afford NOT to plan!

REAL-LIFE SUCCESS STORY

Working with Sarah-Jane has been one of the best decisions I've ever made! Her suggestions make it easy to still eat healthy when life gets busy. Between working, graduate school, and sports, I don't have a lot of extra time to spend thinking about food. Sarah-Jane shows you how to set small goals so the process isn't so overwhelming. These small goals help to achieve your bigger goals. Little changes really can add up! The most valuable thing I learned that I still use all the time is menu planning, dedicating one day to plan your meals for the week and making a grocery list for those meals to be prepared for them. When I'm busy, I already know what the plan is for dinner and don't have to take any more time out of my day to run to the grocery store to get food. Some preparation on the front end gives me more time to do the things I need and want to do. It really is the best time-saver when you're always on the go!

Using Sarah-Jane's tips and tricks, I lost two dress sizes and fifteen pounds, and have kept it off three years later. With her help I was able to change my eating habits and become a much healthier person. It is definitely worth it to spend a little time to invest in your health!

—*Chelsea W.*

TIP FROM CHELSEA: The most important thing Sarah-Jane taught me to remember is that one meal doesn't have to ruin your whole day. If you stray away from your plan at one meal, you can still get back on track with the next one.

Here's How to Plan for Success in Just 30 Minutes

TAKE 10 MINUTES TO:

Use the meal planning tool in Appendix B to plan your whole week's worth of meals. Remember, you can use the menu plan I've already made for you in Chapter 4, or you can create your own meal plan by referring to your meal pattern in Chapter 3 and the pattern portions list (Appendix A).

HERE ARE A FEW KEYS POINTS TO REMEMBER AS YOU SPEND 10 MINUTES PLANNING YOUR MEALS AND SNACKS:

➤ Take a close look at your schedule for the next week. Decide what days you may have more time to cook, and what days you may need to just have leftovers or something else quick on hand, and plan accordingly.

➤ If you are usually out and about in the afternoon when you get hungry for a snack, plan to take some easy snacks with you that don't have to be refrigerated, such as ¼ cup nuts or dried fruit, bananas or apples, or peanut butter and crackers. This may prevent you from hitting the drive-through window or vending machine. (See emergency stash snack list in Chapter 3.)

- Be sure to have a few backups on hand for quick fixes when you're running late, such as sandwich or salad fixings or whole-grain cereal, fruit, and low-fat milk. (See "Plan B" recipes in the recipe collection for more ideas.)
- If you are planning to go out to eat during the week, still plan ahead! Look up nutrition information for menu items. You may be surprised that what you think is the healthiest choice isn't always your best bet.

NEXT, TAKE 5 MINUTES TO:

Plan your grocery store trip by making your grocery list and gathering any coupons you may have. Remember, you can use the grocery lists that I have already put together for you (which coincides with the menu plan I created for you) in Appendix C, or you can make your own list based on the meal plan you created using the blank template from Appendix B.

HERE ARE A FEW KEY THINGS TO REMEMBER AS YOU SPEND THESE 5 MINUTES PREPARING FOR YOUR GROCERY TRIP:

- Make a list every time you go to the grocery store. To save time, arrange the list by area of the store (produce, meats, dairy, canned foods, etc.).
- Gather or download coupons. See the "Quick Couponing" section in Chapter 5 for some ideas on easy, paperless savings.
- Plan to do 80% of your shopping from the perimeter of the store (where most of the healthy foods such as produce, meats, and dairy live) and only 20% from the aisles (where the more packaged and processed foods are found).
- Never go grocery shopping on an empty stomach. If you do, everything will look good, and you'll be more likely to make impulse purchases.

So stop reading and take just 15 minutes to plan for a successful, healthy week ahead. Whenever I don't feel like planning, I think of this quote: "If you fail to plan, you plan to fail!" To save even more time in your planning process, check out the 14-day menu plan in Chapter 4 and the corresponding grocery lists in Appendix C, where I've already done the planning for you!

LAST, AFTER YOU GO TO THE GROCERY STORE, USE YOUR FINAL 15 MINUTES TO:

Preprep some of the food for the week. This will save you worlds of time and enable you to create healthy meals in just minutes on even your busiest days. In Appendix C, I have given you the specific preprep steps for preparing for the week of meals on the meal plan I created.

IF YOU CREATED YOUR OWN MEAL PLAN, YOU MAY WANT TO CONSIDER SOME OF THESE PREPREP STEPS TO GET YOUR WEEK OFF TO A JUMP START.

➤ **Precooking Chicken.** This can be done by deboning a whole chicken or using boneless, skinless chicken breasts. Although using the whole chicken is cheaper, using the breasts is quicker and easier. Simply cook the breasts by baking them in the oven or using some other healthy cooking method, such as boiling, grilling, or roasting (see Chapter 6 for specific instructions on cooking chicken). Chop the chicken, divide it into 2-cup portions (as most casseroles and other chicken dishes call for roughly 2 cups of chicken), and freeze it. Pull it out during the week for use in salads, casseroles, and pastas. The most time-consuming step in chicken dishes is actually cooking the chicken, so this saves you the hassle on those busy nights!

➤ **Precooking Pasta.** Cooking a box of whole wheat pasta at the beginning of the week is an excellent, simple time-saver. Although it's not a difficult task, by the time you bring the water to a boil and cook the pasta, you're talking about at least 20 minutes. When you need a quick lunch or dinner, you will have a healthy base already prepared. And pasta is great, because it can be used in so many ways, from hot spaghetti dishes to cold pasta salads!

- ➤ **Prewashing/Chopping Veggies and Fruit.** After buying fresh produce, take a few minutes to wash it and chop it into bite-size pieces. You'll be more apt to eat fresh, raw veggies and fruit if they are ready to eat (remember, you'll be filling half your plate with fruits and veggies). When you need a quick snack, fruit and veggies will be your first stop instead of calorie-dense snack foods. Also, this advance work will make preparing your meals that much easier.

- ➤ **Doubling Recipes and Freezing.** This tip may seem like common sense, but it's always a winner. Prepare a double batch of your favorite recipe on Sunday night (after your weekly menu planning and grocery shopping are finished), eat a portion of it for dinner, and freeze the leftovers in portion-size containers. This way you can pull it out throughout the week. You may ask, Why freeze it? Why can't I just stick it in the fridge and eat it throughout the week? Well, not only do you risk its spoiling in the fridge if you don't eat it soon enough (most leftovers are unsafe to eat after about four days), but, if you know it's ready to eat in the fridge, you may be likely to overeat. So this freezing method promotes portion control as well!

Since power planning creates a whole new lifestyle for you rather than just another diet, you can expect to see steady success each week. Studies show that the faster you lose weight, the more likely you are to gain it back, plus some. That's why it is important for change to happen at a slow and steady pace. While research is not

A FEW TRICKS TO MAKING FRUITS AND VEGETABLES LAST LONGER

1 If your vegetables come home from the store wet, be sure to pat them dry with paper towels. Then layer them in plastic bags and place them in the crisper section of your refrigerator.

2 As soon as possible after buying, take prewashed leafy greens out of their containers and throw away any bruised or spoiled pieces. Those leaves will spoil the rest!

3 For unwashed greens, separate leaves and rinse them several times in a bowl of ice-cold water with a bit of vinegar or lemon juice to add crispness. If the water starts looking dirty, pour it out and start again with a fresh bowl of ice water. Spin dry if using right away or pat dry with a paper towel, then store in a clean perforated plastic bag in the fridge.

4 Separate fruits from the vegetables. People often toss all the produce into the crisper together, but apples and some other fruits give off ethylene gas, which speeds the ripening of vegetables. Separate your fruits and vegetables so that your veggies don't ripen too fast.

5 Cut off green tops of carrots, turnips, or beets, as the tops draw nutrients out of the roots. Store these vegetables in a cold, dark place that is well ventilated.

6 Keep onions and eggplants out of the refrigerator and store them separately, leaving enough space so air can circulate around them.

7 Tomatoes should remain on the counter to maintain their texture and flavor. Refrigeration may turn tomatoes

(Continued)

mushy. Place them in a bowl lined with a paper towel. Do not keep them near heat sources or direct sunlight.

8 Remove mushrooms from containers and clean them individually with a damp towel. Dry them carefully and store in a paper bag in the fridge.

9 Berries, oranges, pineapples, cherries, grapes, and watermelon do not ripen after picking, so they can go right into the refrigerator. Lemons and limes can be kept on the counter, but they last longer in the refrigerator.

10 Unripe pears, apricots, apples, peaches, plums, mangoes, honeydew melons, cantaloupes, bananas, kiwis, and avocados can soften on the counter. Once they are soft to touch, move them to the refrigerator to halt their ripening.

11 Take bananas apart when you get home from the store. If you leave them connected at the stem, they ripen faster. Keep them on the counter or in a basket with holes, allowing air to circulate. Once bananas are ripe, place them in a plastic bag and put them in the refrigerator. The skin of the banana may turn black from an enzyme reaction, but the cold will halt the ripening of the fruit and keep it from spoiling.

12 Strawberries do best when kept in a paper bag in the fridge. Moisture leads to spoiling of strawberries, so check the bag for dampness every other day.

clear on exactly how long it takes to break bad habits and create good ones, many sources say we need 21 days to a month to make this type of lifestyle change.

The good news is that studies do report that when you replace bad habits with good ones, rather than just trying to quit a bad habit, you are likely to be more successful and make the change much more quickly. That is exactly what the *Schedule Me Skinny* plan provides you with—good habits, like keeping your pantry and fridge stocked with healthy foods to create the "Plan B" meals on busy nights rather than falling into the bad habit of going to the drive-through.

In working with my clients, I have found that how quickly they make these changes really depends on how ready they are to see change in their lives. My guess is that if you are reading this book, you are more than ready not only to lose weight but also to have more control and energy despite your hectic life. With this ready-for-change attitude, you can expect to fully ease into this plan pretty quickly.

Still, I suggest breaking down any lifestyle overhaul into bite-size pieces to make it super easy to achieve. The first week, focus on scheduling your 30-minute power planning session and put it on your calendar. The second week, focus on following the details of your meal plan. The third week, add mindfulness to your eating (as outlined in Chapter 9). By the fourth week, you should have all the pieces put together smoothly, allowing you to lose up to two pounds per week for a total of up to eight pounds in a month.

If you follow the *Schedule Me Skinny* meal pattern, you'll be eating just the right amount of calories from the right balance of foods to lose weight at this steady pace while still consuming enough calories to keep your metabolism and energy levels strong. You will feel good (read: *not starved!*) and be able to keep the weight off. Diets that require very low calorie consumption may lead to quick weight loss, but they also slow the metabolism down and are nearly impossible to stick to.

That's not to say that you'll never have a setback. When you're on a diet, one slipup means you've failed, since diets don't allow any room for setbacks. But this is a lifestyle change, not a diet, and in real life mistakes happen. If you fall back into a bad habit or forget a planning session, it does not mean you have failed. Simply get back to your good habits and planning as soon as you recognize your slipup and you will still succeed. The eight pounds of weight loss per month doesn't happen because of what you do on any single day, but rather because of the new lifestyle you are creating day by day.

Planning is what makes this lifestyle possible, even with a busy schedule, and you can achieve it in just 30 minutes per week. That's a realistic change you can continue to do for the rest of your life. I always tell my clients if they can't follow a diet for the rest of their lives, there is no point in getting on it to start with. If you can't continue to follow a diet, you will just gain all the weight back anyway.

When you start a new lifestyle, it really is life-changing. You can and will continue down this road of power planning, always having a Plan B and keeping the weight off forever!

Believe it or not, after you spend just 30 minutes of power planning, you will be able to create your meals in minutes. You will have the tools at your disposal to create healthy meals and snacks, for the first time. This means that losing weight and eating right will become a reality in your rush-hour-driving, deadline-chasing, social-calendar-filling life. I know because that's my life too, and as much as I'd like to tell you that I grow my own food and prepare a from-scratch dinner worthy of gracing the pages of a nutrition textbook every night, this is the real world, and that simply isn't the case. I have found a way to create satisfying meals from real, whole foods even on my most time-crunched days. And it's easier than you think! Turn the page, and I'll show you how!

CHAPTER 2

BUILDING MEALS AND SNACKS THAT SATISFY

The Schedule Me Skinny plan helps you learn to create meals by following the simple formula for filling your plate that focuses on the right combination of food groups to ensure the right amount of calories, vitamins, and nutrients, as well as flavor.

The Formula for a Balanced Meal

Balance is the key to eating in moderation while feeling satisfied—all without counting calories! You'll load half your plate with fresh, colorful veggies like heirloom tomatoes, sautéed spinach with garlic, or roasted broccoli. Then add satisfying starches like sweet potatoes with dill, nutty quinoa, or sweet golden corn to a quarter of your plate. You'll complete the meal by filling the final fourth of

THE FORMULA FOR A BALANCED MEAL

- Fill half your plate with fruits and/or veggies.
- Fill a quarter of your plate with lean protein.
- Fill a quarter of your plate with a starch.
- Season your meal with healthy fats, herbs, and spices.

your plate with lean protein, like blackened salmon, a perfectly poached egg, or even a juicy steak. Finally, you'll add flavor with healthy fats like nuts or avocado and herbs and spices like rosemary or cumin.

As you can see, unlike a diet, these meals won't leave you disappointed and hungry. My clients often gush when they tell me how this plan doesn't feel like a diet and how satisfied they are with their full plate of food! I remind them the reason it doesn't feel like a diet is because it's not. Eating meals with more foods, not fewer, is a little-known secret to weight loss. Balanced meals provide the nourishment your body needs, while giving your taste buds the flavor they crave. In fact, even as you go from losing weight to maintaining a healthy weight, this formula for creating a balanced meal won't change. In Chapter 10, I will tell you more about the maintenance phase, but rest assured that this balanced meal formula is one you can count on for life.

Filling half your plate with colorful veggies is the easiest way to lose weight without eating less food. Feel free to pile the fresh veggies high, since they are nutrient-rich foods. This means they provide tons of important nutrients like vitamins, minerals, and disease-fighting antioxidants for relatively few calories. Plus, they help fill you up with their high fiber content.

The starches will actually be your secret weapon for warding off those after-dinner munchies. Research shows that when we consume carbohydrates, particularly whole grains, they stimulate our brain to release serotonin, a hormone that helps us feel relaxed and satisfied after a meal. Studies also show that people who eat whole grains have less belly fat than those who don't. I don't know about you, but that sounds like a good reason to enjoy a nice, comforting serving of whole grain pasta. Take that, you depriving low-carb diets! People often shy away from starches because they think that starchy foods like pasta and potatoes are fattening. Actually, they are relatively low in calories because they have a high water content. This high water content makes them filling without being heavy.

Whether you choose a serving of skinless poultry, a lean pork tenderloin or sirloin steak, or even a meatless source such as eggs or beans, lean protein is like the perfect accessory to complete an outfit. Just like your statement necklace takes your little black dress to another level, protein increases the staying power of your meal by filling you up and providing long-lasting energy.

The healthy fats, along with fresh and dried herbs and spices, add the flavor you crave to your meals. There are so many natural, healthy ways to add flavor to your food—after you taste the results, you could never dream of describing them with the word "diet." Nothing can surpass the appetizing aroma of a meal cooking with garlic or rosemary, the creaminess of an avocado, or the savory flavor of extra-virgin olive oil.

Leave out any one of the balanced meal formula components and it will be like pulling the wrong block out of the Jenga tower. Why?

FIRE UP YOUR METABOLISM

When and how often you eat can be just as important as what you eat. Your metabolism is like a fire. If you don't put wood on a fire, after a while the fire burns out. The same thing happens with your metabolism. If you go too long without giving your body fuel, your metabolism burns out (slows down). To keep your metabolism going strong, it is important to eat a meal or snack every four hours. This will also prevent you from making poor choices because you're ravenous. Plus, eating meals and snacks at regularly spaced intervals keeps your blood sugar levels stable, giving you consistent energy throughout the day.

Because each component has a special role in helping you look and feel your best. If you eat too much from any one of these three groups, you will gain weight. But if you eat just the right balance of each group, your body will become more efficient at burning fat, your energy levels will improve, and your body will function at the highest level. If you understand what benefits each group provides, it will be easier to achieve the right balance. Let's take a closer look at each one.

The Power of Protein

Protein is second only to water as the most abundant substance in the human body, so it's easy to see why it's an important component of a healthy diet. Protein is key to building muscle, which helps you look fit and toned. It also helps you stay full after a meal because it takes longer to digest than carbohydrates, and we all know that less mindless snacking means a smaller waistline. One study found that dieters who ate eggs for breakfast lost 65% more weight than those who didn't, even though they ate the same number of calories, probably because the egg breakfasts were higher in filling, quality protein. That's proof for the point that consuming a protein source at each meal is extremely important for weight loss. And if looking younger is on your wish list, protein will help by providing collagen to the connective tissues of the body and to the tissues of the skin, hair, and nails.

When it comes to protein, I suggest eating lean beef once a week, going for a meatless protein day at least once a week, and eating fish at least twice a week. On other days, enjoy lean poultry or lean pork. Fish is an extremely important protein to consume on a weight loss plan, as studies have shown that women who eat fish, especially oily fish like salmon and tuna, two to four times each week have the lowest levels of body fat.

Here are some of the foods rich in protein that you can use to fill a quarter of your plate at each meal (a complete catalog can be found on the pattern portions list [Appendix A]):

➤ Meat (including lean beef and lean pork)
➤ Fish
➤ Poultry (including chicken and turkey, preferably boneless and skinless)
➤ Eggs
➤ Beans
➤ Low-fat milk
➤ Low-fat yogurt (Go for Greek yogurt most often, as it typically has more protein and less sugar. Choose a yogurt with less than 20 grams of sugar per serving.)
➤ Tofu

The Importance of Carbohydrates

Both the colorful fruits and veggies and the starch portions of your plate fall into the carbohydrate food group. Even though some people and diet books would have you believe that carbohydrates are straight from the devil, they play a unique and important role in the body. Carbohydrates offer an immediate source of energy.

Carbohydrates are any foods that contain sugar or starch. This would include:

➤ sweets that contain table sugar (sucrose)
➤ milk and milk products, which contain milk sugar (lactose)
  Note: Although milk products do contain carbohydrates, we are going to count them as proteins for the purpose of our meal pattern, since they have a high protein content.
➤ fruits, which contain fruit sugar (fructose) *Note: Fruits are*

carbohydrates, but they are not starches, so in our balanced meal formula we are including them with vegetables, as they provide many of the same nutrients and benefits as veggies.

➤ starches, which are found in foods made with flour, whole grains, and some vegetables.

I encourage you to focus on the energy-boosting carbs, because they'll make reaching your fitness goals even easier since they take longer than treat carbs to digest, thus helping you feel satisfied with fewer calories. Energy-boosting carbohydrates are also important because they are the primary source of energy for the mind and body. The brain alone requires 100 grams of carbohydrates per day to function at its best. In fact, without enough carbohydrates, you may become deficient in the production of the hormone serotonin and may experience mood swings or depression.

"GOOD" CARBS VS. "BAD" CARBS

○ **Treat Carbohydrates, i.e., "Bad" Carbs:** Moderation is the key here. These treats are okay to enjoy in small quantities as a part of your healthy diet, but they won't provide much sustainable energy or nutrition. Sweets fit into this category, as do some starches, such as processed foods, and anything with added refined sugar or flour, such as white bread, soft drinks, candy, or snack foods.

○ **Energy-Boosting Carbohydrates, i.e., "Good" Carbs:** You want to have at least one of these carbs at every meal, because they provide the long-lasting energy that your body needs. Whole grain foods and starchy veggies fit into this category.

The *Schedule Me Skinny* meal pattern makes it easy to consume the right amount of carbohydrates at each meal to keep your energy levels up and your metabolism burning strong.

Starchy veggies are a particularly good choice, since many of them, such as potatoes, contain a specific type of carbohydrate called resistant starch, which research has shown may promote the burning and shrinking of fat cells! See the pattern portions list (Appendix A) for a complete list of starchy food choices.

Choose a serving of the foods listed below, such as whole grains, beans or legumes, or a starchy veggie, to fill a quarter of your plate at each meal:

1. Whole grains
   - *Whole-wheat breads*
   - *Brown rice or quinoa*
   - *Oatmeal*
   - *Whole-grain cereals*
   - *Other starchy foods, such as granola bars or whole-grain crackers containing a minimum of 3 grams of fiber per 100 calories.*
2. Beans or legumes
3. Starchy vegetables, raw or frozen
   - *Potatoes (sweet potatoes and white potatoes)*
   - *Peas*
   - *Corn*

Avoid or limit the following foods, which contain "treat" carbohydrates:

- *Sugar-sweetened beverages*
- *Candy*
- *Baked goods*
- *Starches made with white flour*

IMPOSTOR WHOLE GRAIN AND WHOLE WHEAT

Some products may claim to be "made with whole grain," or may be called "multi-grain" or "wheat," but still be made primarily with white flour (a simple carbohydrate). Make sure your starches are 100% whole wheat, 100% whole grain, or that the ingredient label lists whole wheat or whole grain as the first ingredient. For example, if a loaf of bread claims to be multi-grain or wheat, but the first ingredient listed is enriched bleached flour (another name for white flour), then it is made primarily from white flour, not whole grains. Instead, find a bread that lists whole-wheat flour as the first ingredient.

Don't panic if some of your favorite foods fit onto the "treat" carb list. The *Schedule Me Skinny* meal pattern includes a daily treat, allowing you to indulge in something you love each day! In fact, research even shows that by having a small treat each day, you can prevent overeating sweets in the long run.

The Abundance of Produce

For the half of your plate that should be filled with colorful fruits and veggies, choose a variety of nonstarchy selections (the more colors on your plate, the more benefits you'll be getting), such as:

- Broccoli
- Carrots
- Tomatoes
- Green beans
- Summer squash
- Asparagus
- Mushrooms
- Spinach
- Salad greens
- Onions
- Peppers

These are just a few of the options, of course. This section can be filled with any of your favorite veggies (that are not listed in the starch section) and any fruits. (A more complete list can be found on the pattern portions list in Appendix A.)

The Fat Factor

By now you know that healthy fats can be used to enhance the flavor of your meals and give them staying power, but fat still gets a bad rap. Let's face it—no one wants to hear her name and the word "fat" used in the same sentence. But fat—once thought of as the ultimate diet sabotage—is actually an essential nutrient that provides long-

THE BEAUTY OF BEANS

If beans are being consumed at a meal that also contains another protein source, they will count as a starch. If they are being consumed at a meal that does not contain another protein source, they will count as your protein. Beans are a natural source of plant protein, but also contain a high amount of carbohydrates. This duality is what makes them versatile. If, for example, you are having a meal of chicken, black beans, cheese, and broccoli, the chicken would count as your protein, the black beans would be your starch, the cheese would be your fat, and of course the broccoli would be your vegetables. Beans are a great choice, as research shows that bean eaters weigh less and have slimmer stomachs than those who do not include beans in their diets.

lasting energy, and when you eat the right type, it can even help you shed pounds.

That's right—fats can play an important role in a healthy diet. They are essential for metabolism and regulation of cellular function, and as a result, it's extremely important to eat them daily in moderation. Not only do they provide satiety, or a sense of fullness, but they also help keep hormones in check and promote the absorption of fat-soluble vitamins A, D, E, and K. However, we all know that a diet in which the fat content is too high can lead to health problems and weight gain. Fats should provide about 20% to 25% of your daily calorie intake, with less than 10% of your calories coming from saturated (solid) fats, found in animal products like fatty cuts of meat and full-fat dairy products like whole milk or butter.

Type and quantity of fat are the two main factors that affect our health. Just as too much fat may be harmful, eating the wrong types of fats may also be detrimental to your overall health. Certain types of fats have health-protective benefits (such as omega-3, mono-unsaturated, and polyunsaturated), while others (saturated and trans) pose some serious health risks. Healthy fats are usually liquid at room temperature and help lower cholesterol levels, support heart and brain health, and reduce inflammation, while unhealthy fats raise cholesterol and increase your risk of heart disease.

TYPES OF DIETARY FAT

➤ **Saturated fat:** When consumed in excess amounts, can lead to high LDL cholesterol (the bad kind) and other heart problems. Limit your intake of foods that are high in saturated fat, such as hydrogenated oils, full-fat dairy products, fatty cuts of meat and fried foods.

➤ **Polyunsaturated fats:** Healthier for the heart and linked with lower levels of LDL cholesterol than saturated fat. You can find polyunsaturated fats in vegetable oils. Within the category of polyunsaturated fats are essential fatty acids, which are associated with better overall health. They include:

> ➤ *Omega-3 fatty acids (highly polyunsaturated): Found in seafood such as tuna, mackerel, and salmon, as well as in walnuts, canola oil, and flaxseed.*

> ➤ *Omega-6 fatty acids (highly polyunsaturated): Found in vegetable oils such as soybean, corn, and safflower.*

➤ **Monounsaturated fats:** Promote heart health by helping to lower LDL cholesterol when substituted for saturated fat, and may also possibly help to raise HDL (good) cholesterol. Research shows that higher intakes

WHAT ABOUT TRANS FATS?

You want to avoid these fats at all costs. They are man-made saturated fats found in processed foods, shortening, and regular stick margarine. "Hydrogenated oils" or "partially hydrogenated oils" appearing in the ingredients list are an indicator that a product contains trans fat. Also, be aware that just because a product has no trans fats does not mean that it has no saturated fat.

MORE BENEFITS OF HEALTHY FATS

Anti-aging benefits don't come just from fruits and veggies. Healthy fats also play a part in keeping us young!

- **Vitamin E:** Found in many healthy fats, including seeds and nuts, this antioxidant is believed to reduce the development of damaged cells that lead to cancer and wrinkles.

  Foods highest in vitamin E include:
    - Wheat germ oil
    - Sunflower seeds
    - Almonds
    - Hazelnuts
    - Peanuts
    - Peanut butter

- **Omega-3 fatty acids:** Antioxidant that is thought to play a role in decreasing inflammation throughout the body, may reduce the risk of stroke, and may even lower the risk of Alzheimer's disease! And there's more good news: in addition to the weight loss and health benefits that all antioxidants offer, studies show that diets rich in omega-3's keep you feeling fuller longer after meals, making weight loss easier. The American Heart Association recommends eating a serving of oily fish, such as salmon, mackerel, herring, lake trout, sardines, or tuna, at least two times a week to get this important nutrient.

  Foods highest in omega-3 fatty acids include:
    - Salmon
    - Mackerel
    - Sardines
    - Halibut
    - Tuna
    - Enriched eggs
    - Flaxseed
    - Walnuts

of monounsaturated fats are associated with lower levels of belly fat. Monounsaturated fats are found in some plant-based oils (such as olive, peanut, canola, and many nut oils), nuts and nut butters, olives and avocados.

When you see "fat" listed on the *Schedule Me Skinny* meal pattern, choose monounsaturated fats most often, followed by poly-unsaturated fats. Choose saturated fats least often and trans fats rarely, if ever. Your pattern portions list (Appendix A) will tell you what foods fall into which fat category. It also lists appropriate portion sizes of different fats.

Whew! That was a lot of information. But don't get freaked out! You need to understand the components of healthy eating to appreciate how simple this plan makes it. Feel free to go back to this section whenever you would like, but I promise, you do NOT have to memorize any of this. In fact, it will soon make a lot more sense, because now I'm going to show you how easy it is to build a balanced breakfast, lunch, or dinner using these food groups. All you have to remember is four simple steps.

Four Steps to Creating a Flavorful, Balanced Meal
That's all you have to remember!

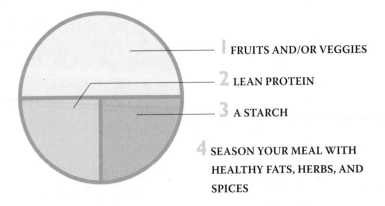

1 FRUITS AND/OR VEGGIES

2 LEAN PROTEIN

3 A STARCH

4 SEASON YOUR MEAL WITH HEALTHY FATS, HERBS, AND SPICES

CHAPTER 3

YOUR *SCHEDULE ME SKINNY* MEAL PATTERN

Wondering how you are going to put all of this together? Don't sweat it! I have created a 14-day menu plan, complete with grocery lists, that will easily fit into your busy life. The meal pattern puts together the three concepts of balanced eating that we've been talking about—filling half your plate with fruits and/or veggies, filling a quarter of your plate with lean protein, filling a quarter of your plate with a starch, and seasoning your meal with healthy fats, herbs, and spices—and creates a fill-in-the-blank format for actual breakfasts, lunches, and dinners that you can eat with confidence. Use this balanced meal pattern below for the times you'd like to build your own meals.

Each meal on the *Schedule Me Skinny* meal pattern and menu plan is broken down into the components of the essential food groups your body needs, in the proper proportions to create the total number of calories you need per day to lose weight without feeling hungry or slowing your metabolism down. You can use the meal pattern like a checklist, making sure you get all the listed components at each meal. If you do this, you won't even have to worry about calorie counting because, as you can see on the pattern, I've already done that for you.

You will also see that the calories are spaced fairly evenly throughout the day. There are many nutrients—protein and calcium, for instance—that can be absorbed only in limited amounts at any given time. Balancing the calories throughout the day also means nutrients are delivered to your body so that you can get maximum benefits from them.

You'll also shed pounds when you eat consistently throughout the day, because that pace prevents blood sugar spikes and crashes, which can lead to fat storage. It also promotes a fast metabolism because you are giving your body just the right amount of fuel to burn at any given time.

I provided the calories on the meal pattern for each meal and snack as a reference point, not because you have to count them. As you navigate your busy schedule with lots of food options thrown at you, you'll need to make choices about what's worth eating. It's like when you go shopping—you may not know down to the cent how much money is in your bank account, but you do have a general idea of how much you can spend. So with your new healthy lifestyle in place, when you see a food that contains 500 calories, you'll have a reference point to decide if you really want to spend roughly a third of your daily calories on that one thing. You can skip the guesswork and turn right to the menu plan later in Chapter 4 to chow down on the meals I've already created especially for you, or you can create your own meals by referring to the pattern portion list (Appendix A) to determine what foods fit into each food group listed and what counts as a serving for each one. The list will allow you to mix and

WHEN YOU SHOULD EAT WHAT

1 Spread your calories evenly throughout the day. Recent research published in the *International Journal of Obesity* found that people who ate the majority of their calories later in the day had a slower weight-loss rate and lost significantly less weight than early eaters!

2 Don't forget to include a good source of protein for breakfast! Current studies show that having a protein-rich breakfast significantly improves appetite control and reduces unhealthy snacking on high-fat or high-sugar foods in the evening.

3 Include good sources of whole grains at the dinner table. Recent research suggests there is an advantage in concentrating carbohydrate intake in the evening, especially for people at risk of developing diabetes or cardiovascular disease due to obesity. Studies showed that individuals who ate the majority of their carbohydrates at dinner experienced increased satiety and reduced risk of diabetes and cardiovascular disease.

match foods within each food group and make the pattern work for you whether you are cooking at home, eating out with friends, or enjoying a home-cooked meal with your extended family. The list also allows you to be creative with your cooking. As you try the recipes in the recipe collection, you can use foods you already have in your fridge and pantry to make substitutions in the recipes to tailor them to your liking. For example, if you like rice instead of pasta, feel free to switch these ingredients. And if you're not a fan of pork, try substituting chicken or beans.

The Meal Pattern

BREAKFAST (350 Calories)	**EXAMPLE**
1 serving starch	1 100% whole-wheat English muffin
1 serving protein	1 container (6 oz.) low-fat yogurt
1 serving fat	1 tbsp. peanut butter
1 serving fruits/vegetables	1 cup blueberries

LUNCH (450 Calories)	
2 servings fruits/vegetables	2 cups salad greens with carrots and tomatoes
1 serving protein	5 oz. grilled chicken
1 serving fat	2 tbsp. light salad dressing
1 serving starch	6 whole-grain crackers, such as Triscuits

DINNER (450 Calories)	
1 serving protein	5 oz. sirloin steak
1 serving fat	1 tbsp. vegetable oil–based butter spread
1 serving starch	½ large baked potato (fist-size)
2 servings fruits/vegetables	½ cup steamed broccoli and 1 tomato, sliced

SNACK (200 Calories)	
1 serving fruits/vegetables or starch	1 medium apple
1 serving protein or fat	1 piece string cheese

TREAT (150 Calories)
2 fun-size candy bars or one 12-oz. sweetened drink

Building Breakfast

Let's start with breakfast.

Ideally you should eat breakfast within an hour and a half of waking. Wait any longer, and your body may think it's not getting any fuel and switch to starvation mode, which puts your metabolism in slo-mo, interfering with your body's fat-burning ability.

Skipping breakfast is one of the worst things you can do. Breakfast helps to jump-start your metabolism and energy for the day. Plus, if you eat a balanced breakfast it can prevent overeating later in the day and promote weight loss. In fact, a study from Virginia Commonwealth University in Richmond found that obese women who ate a high-calorie breakfast shed about 40 pounds in eight months, but those who ate a low-calorie breakfast experienced a loss of only about 9 pounds.

If you do nothing else, please, please, please don't skip breakfast! Is it worth being late to work if it would mean that you look amazing in your LBD this weekend? Then eat breakfast. No. Matter. What. That's not to say that some days it won't be challenging to find time to eat breakfast. We all oversleep sometimes or have the occasional outfit crisis. That's why it's important to have some quick breakfast ideas that are healthy grab-and-go options.

Remember, all you need is the four essential components of a healthy meal to create the perfect breakfast that is balanced and filling. No cooking required!

Each breakfast you eat should be about 350 calories and include one serving of starch, one serving of protein, at least one serving of a fruit or veggie, and some healthy fat. You can check out the pattern portions list (Appendix A) for serving sizes for specific foods, or you can enjoy the breakfast ideas I've created and already balanced out for you on the menu plan. If you need to add a little sweetness to your breakfast to make it more appetizing, go ahead. In fact, you'll see that many of the breakfasts in the recipe collection contain a

GRAB-AND-GO BREAKFASTS!

1 **Almond Butter and Banana Waffle Sandwich:** Toast 2 whole-grain frozen waffles (such as Van's). Spread one of the waffles with 1 tablespoon almond butter, ½ sliced banana, and a dash of cinnamon. Top with the other waffle and consume!

2 **Berry Granola Parfait:** Layer 6 ounces plain, nonfat Greek yogurt, 1 cup fresh berries, ¼ cup store-bought granola (look for brands with about 120 calories per serving), and 1 tablespoon honey in a mason jar or Tupperware container. Drizzle with honey and enjoy!

3 **Mango Tango Spinach Smoothie:** Combine 1 cup skim milk, 1 sliced banana, ½ cup chopped frozen mango, 1 tablespoon ground flaxseed, 1 cup fresh spinach, ¼ cup plain nonfat Greek yogurt, and 2 teaspoons honey. Blend until smooth. *Tip:* Make it without wasting your precious morning minutes by washing the spinach and slicing the banana the night before. Then put all ingredients (except for the milk, yogurt and honey) in a zip-top bag and stash in the freezer. In the morning, all you'll have to do is throw the ingredients in the blender, and you're good to go.

4 **Easy Egg Fiesta Wrap:** Pour ¼ cup liquid 100% egg whites into a small bowl sprayed with nonstick cooking spray. Microwave in 30-second intervals until cooked through. Spread ¼ avocado on a 100% whole wheat tortilla (pick one that has 150 calories or less). Top with eggs, ½ cup chopped spinach, 2 tablespoons salsa, and ¼ cup shredded cheese.

5 **Peanut Butter Banana Flax Oatmeal:** Microwave 1 packet unflavored instant oatmeal with ¾ cup skim milk and ½ mashed banana. Top cooked mixture with 1 tablespoon natural peanut butter, 1 tablespoon ground flaxseed, and 1 teaspoon brown sugar.

SKIP THE MIDMORNING MUNCHIES

One snack time you might want to skip is midmorning. A 2011 study from the *Journal of the American Dietetic Association* found that dieters who noshed between breakfast and lunch tended to snack later in the day too. This seemed to be an obstacle to their weight loss, as morning snackers lost 4% less weight in a year than did those who didn't snack between breakfast and lunch. If you follow your meal pattern to consume a balanced breakfast and eat lunch within four hours after breakfast, skipping a midmorning snack shouldn't be a problem.

little honey or even dark chocolate! That's because recent research found that people who ate a breakfast that included a little something sweet lost more weight and kept it off better than those who ate low-carb, low-calorie breakfasts. Breakfast just got a lot more exciting!

Building Lunch and Dinner

You can probably guess what comes next. For lunch and dinner, you'll want to include the same four components to keep all your meals balanced.

Brown-bagging it is the easiest way to ensure balance at lunch. Bringing your lunch to work will not only help you avoid calorie-laden restaurant meals but can also save you up to $3,000 a year! And bringing lunch from home does not have to be time-consuming or boring. Save the moola for your after-weight-loss wardrobe and check out my super-easy lunch ideas.

Lunch should be 450 calories and include one serving of starch,

BROWN BAG LUNCH!

1 **Greek Avocado Veggie Salad:** Combine ¼ avocado, cubed, with ½ cup chickpeas, ½ cup diced cucumber, and ½ cup diced tomatoes. Top with 2 tablespoons crumbled Feta cheese. For the dressing, whisk together 1 tablespoon olive oil, 1½ tablespoons red wine vinegar, a dash of dried oregano, a dash of dried basil, and salt and pepper to taste. Toss salad and dressing. Serve over a bed of spinach with a cup of grapes on the side.

Tip: To avoid soggy salad, pack the dressing in a separate container and toss with the salad just before eating.

2 **Taco Salad:** Combine 1 cup chopped romaine, ½ cup black beans, ¼ cup chopped tomatoes, and 2 tablespoons shredded Mexican-style cheese. Toss with 1 tablespoon olive oil, 1½ tablespoons lime juice, a small squirt of honey, and salt and pepper to taste. Pair with ½ cup blueberries and 2 tablespoons almonds for some crunch.

3 **Nutty Quinoa Salad with Strawberries:** Combine ½ cup cooked quinoa with ½ cup chopped strawberries, 1 cup chopped spinach, 2 tablespoons sunflower seeds, 1 ounce crumbled goat cheese, and a few torn basil leaves. Serve with 10 baby carrots and 2 tablespoons hummus.

4 **Tuna, Lettuce, and Tomato:** Mix 1 5-ounce can tuna (drained) with 1 tablespoon light mayonnaise and 3 table-spoons nonfat Greek yogurt. Season with salt and pepper to taste. Spread on a slice of 100% whole-wheat bread. Top with 1 piece romaine lettuce and 2 tomato slices, then another piece of bread. Pair with an apple for a complete lunch.

one serving of protein, at least two servings of fruits/veggies, and some healthy fat. While there is no minimum amount of time to wait between breakfast and lunch, make sure you eat lunch no more than four hours after breakfast to prevent overeating and to keep your blood sugar levels and metabolism in check. Other than the four-hour rule, just let your hunger be your guide in deciding when to take your lunch break. Check out the tips in Chapter 9 about distinguishing true, physical hunger from emotional hunger.

Your dinner should also be 450 calories and include the same components as your lunch. Remember that you should either eat your dinner within four hours after your lunch or have a snack in the afternoon if it will be more than four hours between your meals.

When it comes to dinner, cooking is always my first choice. I love cooking. I really do. But to be real with you, I must confess that some days I am just too busy and tired by dinnertime to start preparing a balanced meal from scratch. The good news for me and anyone else who leads a busy life is that there are more and more healthy options these days when it comes to convenient prepared foods, such as frozen meals. But not all these meals are healthy, so it helps to have some criteria to use when deciding which convenience food you should put in your grocery cart.

First, take a look at the ingredients list. Ingredients lists start with what the product contains the most of and progress to what the product contains the least of. Look for fruits, veggies, whole grains, and/or lean proteins at the top of the list. Then check out the nutrition facts panel. Stick with frozen meals that have these characteristics: between 300 and 450 calories; no more than 3½ grams saturated fat; no more than 33% daily value sodium; at least 4–5 grams fiber; and includes vegetables. If the frozen meal you choose is under your calorie allotment for that meal and doesn't have 2 servings of veggies/ fruit, add a piece of fresh fruit or a veggie (remember to fill half your plate with fruits and veggies).

Smart Snacking

We can't talk about eating in a balanced way without mentioning snacks. You have one snack per day as a part of your meal pattern, and you can choose when you would like to eat it. To get the best benefit from your snack, follow these tips for smart snacking:

➤ If you are working out intensely for an hour or more, you may want to have your daily snack after your workout. This will help your body refuel and help your muscles rebuild, provided your snack contains the recommended combination of carbohydrates and protein.

➤ Any time you have a gap between meals that lasts four hours or more, you should have your snack time during that gap. This will help prevent overeating and keep your energy levels up. Make sure to always keep a healthy snack in your car or purse just in case you end up having a longer gap between meals than you were planning on (see the "Top 10 Emergency Snacks" breakout box for ideas).

➤ If you eat an early dinner and stay up late, or if you have trouble sleeping at night, you may want to have your snack before bed. No matter what you may have heard, there is no "curfew" on when you should stop eating to promote weight loss. However, what you choose to snack on (and the amount of it) at night is super important.

SMART BEDTIME SNACKS

1. ¼ bag unbuttered popcorn with a 6-ounce container low-fat yogurt
2. 1 slice whole-wheat bread with 2 tablespoons all-fruit spread
3. 1 cup oatmeal prepared with water with ½ small banana, sliced
4. 5 whole-grain crackers with 1 piece string cheese
5. 1 slice whole-wheat toast with 1 tablespoon almond butter
6. ¾ cup whole-grain Cheerios with 1 cup skim milk
7. ¼ cup sunflower seeds
8. 2 tablespoons almonds with 2 tablespoons raisins
9. ¼ cup 1% low-fat cottage cheese with ½ cup peaches
10. 1 tablespoon peanut butter with 1 small apple, sliced

Let's be real—you won't always be in your kitchen with access to fresh fruit and veggies when the munchies hit. If you find yourself ravenous between meals when you're out and about, you need to have a plan. Otherwise, you will get so hungry that you'll eat anything you can get your hands on, even that calorie-bomb candy bar or those salt-laden chips from the convenience store or the office vending machine.

Keep an emergency snack stash in your car or purse, with healthy eats that don't require refrigeration. These snacks should still fit into your *Schedule Me Skinny* snack guidelines of 200 calories and be a combination of carbs or fruit or veggies plus a healthy fat or protein. If you need some ideas for getting your stash started, check out the box below.

TOP 10 EMERGENCY SNACKS STASH

1 ¼ cup dried apricots mixed with 2 tablespoons pumpkin seeds

2 2.6-ounce tuna packet with six 100% whole grain crackers (such as Triscuits)

3 Nutty popcorn trail mix: In a baggie, combine 2 tablespoons almonds + 2 tablespoons dried cranberries + 2 cups air-popped popcorn

4 1 small banana with 1 tablespoon almond or peanut butter (look for single-serving packets)

5 4-ounce unsweetened applesauce cup with ¼ cup sunflower seeds

6 Lean beef jerky (single-serving pack) and 1 small apple

(Continued)

7 I cup carrot sticks, I-ounce serving Snyder's Whole-Wheat Pretzel Sticks, and a wedge of Laughing Cow cheese. If you will be eating your snack in less than four hours, this snack works as a portable option, since these items can stay unrefrigerated just fine for about that long. If it is going to be longer than that, or if you would like to be able to take more fresh options with you, simply get a small cooler with ice packs to keep in your car.

8 Snack bars: Choose bars with a combination of carbohydrates and protein, with less than 200 calories and at least 3 grams of fiber, such as Luna bars. I always keep one of these in my gym bag and my purse.

9 One rice cake with Horizon Organic Low-fat Chocolate Milk, 8-ounce box: If you are craving something sweet on the go, this snack is a great option. These milk boxes are shelf-stable (meaning they don't need refrigeration until after they are opened), and they pair nicely with a whole-grain rice cake for a snack that is a good source of calcium and also provides a little protein and fiber.

10 One 100-calorie packet almonds and a single-serving bag freeze-dried fruit (100 calories or less).

Treats

There is really only one "rule" when it comes to your daily treat. It just has to stay within your 150-calorie treat budget. As far as what the treat is, that is totally up to you! It can be anything that you love or are craving that day. Want a soda? Go for it! Craving chips? Indulge. Just check the nutrition label and make sure you enjoy the correct serving size to stay within 150 calories, and you are good to go! You can also use your treat calories to add an extra serving of something you love to a meal. For instance, if you can't resist the bread basket at your favorite restaurant, you could choose to use your treat calories the day you go there to savor a roll.

I don't recommend saving up your treat calories all week and using them all on one day, however, because this defeats the purpose of having a daily treat so that you won't binge at a later time. Also, that mentality destroys the balance we are trying to achieve of evenly spacing your calories throughout each day and each week to keep your metabolism and blood sugar levels at a steady place. So take the time each day to treat yourself to something you truly want, and you will feel alive, not deprived!

If you would like to make your treat do double duty by satisfying a craving and providing some benefits, take a look at the possibilities below to have your cake and eat it too!

150-CALORIE TREATS WITH BENEFITS

1 **Strawberries and Dark Chocolate:** Five large strawberries + 1 ounce dark chocolate. Strawberries are great sources of vitamin C and manganese. Look for dark chocolate with a cocoa content of 70% or more and watch the portion size! Stick to about 1 ounce of chocolate. Quality dark chocolate in moderation may help reduce high blood pressure and LDL (bad cholesterol).

2 **Parmesan Garlic Popcorn:** 3 cups air-popped popcorn + ½ teaspoon extra-virgin olive oil + 2½ teaspoons Parmesan + 1 teaspoon garlic powder. Popcorn has more antioxidants than most vegetables! Take this great snack, and instead of packing on the calories and fat with butter, sprinkle with olive oil, Parmesan, and garlic powder!

(Continued)

3 **Store-bought Dark Chocolate–Covered Almonds:** This great grab-and-go treat has not only the health benefits of dark chocolate but also those of almonds, which are packed with vitamin E and have four to five times more antioxidants than most other nuts. Careful with the portion sizes! A one-ounce serving is about the size of a shot glass.

4 **Banana Ice Cream:** For one serving, freeze 1½ medium diced bananas and simply toss them in the blender until smooth. You get the creamy sweet "ice cream," without the saturated fat and calories!

5 **Angel Food Cake Topped with Berries:** 1 slice cake (1 ounce) + 1 cup mixed berries. Take this low-fat dessert, throw on a serving of fruit, and you'll have an indulgent yet light treat. Choose blueberries and strawberries for the cardiovascular benefits. Recent research showed that women who ate at least three servings of blueberries or strawberries per week had fewer heart attacks.

6 **Whole-Wheat Cinnamon Toast:** Sugar, spice, and everything nice comes with this lovely treat. Toast a slice of whole grain bread and top with 1 teaspoon butter, ½ teaspoon brown sugar, and as much cinnamon as your heart desires! This snack is a great source of whole grains, and research shows that cinnamon may help to lower LDL (bad cholesterol) and regulate blood sugar!

7 **Frozen California Grapes:** 1¼ cups grapes. Throw a vine in the freezer for a few hours, and you will have a cool, delicious treat packed with antioxidants and other nutrients. Grapes contain resveratrol, which studies indicate may promote blood vessel health and help lower levels of LDL cholesterol.

8 **Greek Frozen Yogurt Drops:** Combine ½ cup nonfat plain Greek yogurt with 1 cup frozen berries and 1 teaspoon honey. Line a baking sheet with parchment paper and drop ¼ teaspoons of the mixture onto the sheet. Freeze for a few hours until solid and pour all the drops into a plastic baggie. Store in the freezer until you want to enjoy! This snack is an excellent source of high-fiber fruit and low-fat dairy.

9 **Strawberry Milk Shake:** Rich in nutrients, such as vitamin C, and antioxidants, for which strawberries are known. Combine 1 cup skim milk with ¾ cup frozen, hulled strawberries and ½ tablespoon honey. Blend until smooth.

10 **Cubed Mangoes Dusted with Cinnamon:** Combine 1½ cups mangoes with 2 teaspoons cinnamon. Mangoes, with just under 3 grams of fiber per cup, are a very satisfying snack. The cinnamon adds a warm, satisfying flavor.

11 **Hot Chocolate:** Add 3 tablespoons cocoa powder and a pinch of stevia to 1 cup heated skim milk, then dab on 1 tablespoon fat-free whipped topping. This healthy, warm treat trumps the premixed varieties, which often contain artificial sweeteners and trans fats.

CHAPTER 4

YOUR 14-DAY SCHEDULE ME SKINNY MENU

I hope you are hungry, because this 14-day meal plan is chock-full of the deliciously slimming, healthy foods you've been reading about. Find the recipes for meals in italics on your meal plan in the recipe collection following Chapter 10. Suggested side items are listed after the semicolon.

Use the plan as is to get started with 14 days of healthy meal ideas, or mix and match meals based on your mood. I have already done the math for you—each breakfast is right around 350 calories, while each lunch and dinner is about 450 calories and snacks come in at about 200 calories each. I have made suggestions for your daily treat, but you can have whatever your heart desires, from a gourmet coffee drink to a bag of chips, provided that you stay within the 150-calories-per-day treat budget.

Remember, when your day doesn't go as planned, you can substitute a lunch or dinner on this meal plan with a super-easy Plan B meal (read more about Plan B meals) from the recipe section. Just use the Plan B grocery list that appears in Appendix C to stock your pantry and freezer before you get started with the *Schedule Me Skinny* plan.

I have also included separate grocery lists for each week of the 14-day plan in Appendix C to make your weekly power planning sessions even faster.

Let the weight loss and feeling great begin!

Week 1 Menu

MONDAY

Breakfast: Apple Cinnamon Breakfast Pizza; 1 (12 oz.) nonfat latte

Lunch: Nutty Quinoa Salad with Strawberries; 10 baby carrots with 2 tbsp. hummus

Snack: Loaded Banana

Dinner: 2 *Black Jack Tacos*; carrot and pepper "fries": 2 cups baby carrots and 1 large bell pepper (sliced) sprayed with cooking spray, sprinkled with a dash of chili powder, roasted at 400° F for 20–25 minutes until slightly tender

Treat: Strawberries and Dark Chocolate

TUESDAY

Breakfast: On-the-Go Omelet; 1 slice whole-wheat toast, 1 medium banana

Lunch: Italian-Style Loaded Baked Potato; 2 cups baby spinach

with ½ cup chopped tomatoes, 1 cup baby carrots, 1 cup
sliced mushrooms, and 2 tbsp. light salad dressing

Snack: *Nutty Choco Popcorn*

Dinner: *Sarah-Jane and Joe's Blackened Salmon*; salad made
with 3 cups spinach, ½ cup sliced strawberries, ½ cup sliced
apples, and 2 tbsp. light salad dressing; 1 slice whole-wheat
bread, toasted and topped with 1 tsp. butter

Treat: 1¼ cups frozen grapes

WEDNESDAY

Breakfast: *Peanut Butter Banana Flax Oatmeal*

Lunch: Leftovers: Leftover *Blackened Salmon* fillet on 2 slices
whole-wheat bread with 1 Bibb lettuce leaf, 1 slice tomato,
and mustard (optional); 1 cup fresh strawberries

Snack: 2 tbsp. dry-roasted almonds with 1 tbsp. raisins

Dinner: 1 serving *Mediterranean Quinoa Bowl*

Treat: *Banana Ice Cream*

THURSDAY

Breakfast: *Easy Egg Fiesta Wrap*; 1 medium banana

Lunch: Leftovers: Leftover serving *Mediterranean Quinoa Bowl*

Snack: 1 medium sliced apple with 1 tbsp. peanut butter

Dinner: *Portabella Pizzas*; ½ cup chickpeas, ¼ cup chopped
tomatoes tossed with ½ cup cooked quinoa seasoned with
salt, pepper, and garlic powder

Treat: *Whole-Wheat Cinnamon Toast*

FRIDAY

Breakfast: *Apple Cinnamon Breakfast Pizza*; 1 (12 oz.) nonfat
latte

Lunch: *Tuna, Lettuce, and Tomato Sandwich*; 1 cup fresh
strawberries
Snack: ½ cup low-fat cottage cheese with 1 cup grapes
Dinner: Night Out: Applebee's: Napa Chicken and Portabellos
with the sides it comes with (sautéed zucchini, peppers,
mushrooms, and red potatoes)
Treat: McDonald's ice cream cone on the way home from
Applebee's

SATURDAY

Breakfast: *Peanut Butter and Banana Waffle Sandwich*
Lunch: *Salmon and Chickpea Lettuce Wraps*; 1 cup steam-in-
the-bag frozen mixed seasoned veggies
Snack: *2 Angel Eggs*
Dinner: *Roast Beef Melt*
Treat: 1 oz. (a shot glass full) store-bought dark-chocolate-
covered almonds

SUNDAY

Breakfast: *Berry Granola Parfait*
Lunch: Leftovers: *Roast Beef Melt*
Snack: ½ cup grapes and 3 tbsp. dry-roasted almonds
Dinner: Night Out: Olive Garden: Linguine alla Marinara (ask
for the lunch portion) with 1 serving Garden Fresh Salad
(with Dressing)
Treat: 1 breadstick with dinner at Olive Garden

Week 2 Menu

MONDAY

Breakfast: Ooey-Gooey Strawberry Chocolate Chip Oatmeal

Lunch: Lentil Stuffed Peppers; 1 single serving steam-in-the-microwave-container frozen veggies, and ½ cup cooked quinoa

Snack: ¼ cup hummus with 1 cup assorted raw veggies

Dinner: 2 *Black Jack Tacos*; carrot and pepper "fries": 2 cups baby carrots and 1 large bell pepper (sliced) sprayed with cooking spray, sprinkled with a dash of chili powder, roasted at 400° F for 20–25 minutes until slightly tender

Treat: Starbucks Tall Caramel Frappuccino Light

TUESDAY

Breakfast: Berry Granola Parfait

Lunch: Lunch Out: Panera Bread: Ask for their Secret Menu Power Steak Lettuce Wrap with a Whole-Grain Baguette and an apple

Snack: 1 banana with 2 tbsp. dry-roasted almonds

Dinner: Slow-Cooker Mediterranean Chicken; ½ cup cooked quinoa mixed with 1 cup spinach sautéed in 1 tsp. olive oil, 2 tbsp. goat cheese, and 2 tbsp. sun-dried tomatoes (make double portions of the sides for lunch tomorrow)

Treat: Strawberry Milkshake

WEDNESDAY

Breakfast: Easy Egg Fiesta Wrap; 1 medium banana

Lunch: Leftovers: Leftover *Slow-Cooker Mediterranean Chicken*; leftover sides: ½ cup cooked quinoa mixed with

1 cup spinach sautéed in 1 tsp. olive oil, 2 tbsp. goat cheese, and 2 tbsp. sun-dried tomatoes

Snack: 1 slice whole-grain toast topped with 1 tbsp. peanut butter

Dinner: Dinner Out: Ruby Tuesday: Hickory Bourbon Chicken with Creamy Mashed Cauliflower and Sugar Snap Peas

Treat: Cubed Mangoes Dusted with Cinnamon

THURSDAY

Breakfast: Peanut Butter and Banana Waffle Sandwich

Lunch: Tuna, Lettuce, and Tomato Sandwich; 1 cup fresh strawberries

Snack: 3 cups air-popped popcorn sprinkled with ¼ cup shredded cheese

Dinner: Mini Meat Loaves; 1 small baked potato with 2 tbsp. plain nonfat Greek yogurt, 2 tbsp. shredded cheese; and 2 cups sliced zucchini sprayed with cooking spray, seasoned with salt, roasted at 400° F for 20 minutes (make double potato and zucchini for lunch tomorrow)

Treat: Berries and Whip Cream Parfait

FRIDAY

Breakfast: Peanut Butter and Berry Yogurt; 1 slice whole-wheat toast

Lunch: Leftovers: *Mini Meat Loaves*; 1 small baked potato with 2 tbsp. plain nonfat Greek yogurt, 2 tbsp. shredded cheese; and 2 cups sliced zucchini sprayed with cooking spray, seasoned with salt, roasted at 400° F for 20 minutes

Snack: 2 tbsp. raisins and 2 tbsp. dry-roasted almonds

Dinner: No-Mess Baked Fish and Veggies

Treat: Hot Chocolate

SATURDAY

Breakfast: On-the-Go Omelet; 1 slice whole-wheat toast, 1 medium banana

Lunch: Leftovers: Leftover *No-Mess Baked Fish and Vegetables*

Snack: 1 container (6 oz.) nonfat Greek yogurt topped with 1 cup berries

Dinner: Pan-Glazed Chicken with Kale and Basil; Slow-Cooker Sweet Potatoes; 1 large tomato, sliced

Treat: 1 oz. (a shot glass full) store-bought dark-chocolate-covered almonds

SUNDAY

Breakfast: Apple Cinnamon Breakfast Pizza; 1 (12 oz.) nonfat latte

Lunch: Leftovers: Leftover *Pan-Glazed Chicken with Kale and Basil; Slow-Cooker Sweet Potatoes*; 1 large tomato, sliced

Snack: Fresh Goat Cheese Bruschetta

Dinner: Portabella Pizzas; ½ cup black beans, ¼ cup chopped tomatoes tossed with ½ cup cooked quinoa seasoned with salt, pepper, and garlic powder

Treat: Chocolate Avocado Pudding

Plan B Meals

With busy schedules and lots of demands on your time, you should always have a Plan B ready. Stock your pantry and fridge with these staples and you'll be able to throw together a healthy and quick dinner on super-busy days. If you stock up on these items at the beginning of the month, you'll be good to go.

Pantry Must-Haves	Freezer Must-Haves
Whole-wheat pasta	Berries
Canned, diced chicken breast, packed in water	Broccoli, corn, peas, edamame, green beans, peppers, mixed veggies, spinach
Microwavable brown rice or quinoa	Veggie burgers (such as Chipotle Black Bean made by MorningStar Farms)
Fresh sweet potatoes	Nuts (such as almonds, pecans, and pine nuts)
Corn tortillas	Fish that can be cooked from frozen, such as Gorton's Classic Grilled Salmon
Beans (black, chickpeas, kidney)	100-calorie 100% whole-wheat sandwich thins
Canned fruit/veggies, such as pineapple in its own juice, diced and crushed tomatoes, corn	Red and yellow onions
Canned wild salmon and chunk light tuna, packed in water	
Lower sodium vegetable/chicken broth	
Parmesan cheese (may require refrigeration after opening)	
Dried cherries, raisins, cranberries	
Instant oatmeal	
Salsa (may require refrigeration after opening)	
Sun-dried tomatoes (may require refrigeration after opening)	
Citrus fruit (such as lemons and limes)	
Standard-size baked tortilla chips (140 calories per ounce)	

With these staples, I create all kinds of yummy dishes, from flavorful Chipotle Grilled Salmon with Pineapple Salsa to a quick Veggie Burger with Sweet Potato Fries. You'll find these go-to recipes in the "Plan B Meals" part of the recipe collection. There's always time for a healthy meal even if your day doesn't go as planned!

Why This Meal Pattern Works

I created this meal pattern and menu plan for you with both weight loss and health in mind. While it is true that if you eat fewer calories than you burn, you will lose weight, not all calories are created equal. For instance, a piece of salmon may have more calories than a piece of candy, but the salmon also has a wealth of nutrients that your body needs to stay healthy while the candy has virtually none. When your body is healthy, it functions at its best, allowing your metabolism to work at full speed to use calories efficiently and to burn fat. When you are unhealthy from eating an unbalanced diet or not getting enough of the nutrients you need, your body has to use energy to try and nourish or repair itself. This could even lead to your body breaking down lean, fat-burning muscle for fuel. Eating a nutrient-rich, balanced diet provides the fuel your body needs to stay healthy and keep its energy focused on using calories correctly and burning fat.

The foods I recommend in your meal pattern and feature in the recipe collection not only help you shed pounds, but they also add years to your life! Incorporating these nutrient-dense foods into your meal plan can make you both feel and look younger!

The fruits and veggies that should fill half your plate contain antioxidants, which combat nasty free radicals in the body in order to prevent harsh effects on our health and appearance! Free radicals can lead to cell damage, which can cause aging and disease. You won't see the effects of cell damage immediately, but they will creep up on you in the form of wrinkles, poor vision, impaired hearing, and chronic disease. Not to mention inflammation, which is also associated with being overweight or obese. There's good news,

MORE ON ANTIOXIDANTS

Carotenoids are a group of antioxidants abundant in fruits and vegetables, which include beta-carotene, lycopene, lutein, and zeaxanthin.

- **Lutein and zeaxanthin:** These two antioxidants may keep skin looking young and help to prevent vision loss as we age.

    Foods highest in both lutein and zeaxanthin include:
    - Dark green leafy vegetables
    - Egg yolks
    - Yellow and orange fruits and vegetables

- **Beta-carotene:** Found abundantly in orange-colored fruits and vegetables such as mangoes, squash, carrots, and sweet potatoes, beta-carotene has been associated with better memory performance. Plus, you can revitalize your skin with this anti-aging antioxidant, as it increases cell turnover and promotes new skin cell growth.

    Foods highest in beta-carotene include:
    - Carrots and carrot juice
    - Canned pumpkin
    - Sweet potatoes
    - Spinach

- **Lycopene:** This age-fighting antioxidant is associated with prevention of heart disease, elevated cholesterol, and cancer. Lycopene along with beta-carotene also protects against UV damage to the skin, the number one cause of wrinkles.

    Foods highest in lycopene include:

- Tomatoes, tomato juice, tomato sauce, and tomato ketchup
- Watermelon
- Pink grapefruit

○ **Vitamin C:** This antioxidant does more than just boost your immune system. It also helps to protect your skin from UV damage and can even help skin recover from previous sun damage, since it promotes collagen production, which keeps skin looking silky smooth.

Foods highest in vitamin C include:
- Red bell peppers
- Yellow bell peppers
- Strawberries
- Broccoli
- Orange juice

Polyphenols are a class of phytochemicals or plant-based chemicals that act as antioxidants in the body.

○ **Anthocyanins:** This type of polyphenol is found in brightly colored fruits such as berries and has potent antioxidant/anti-inflammatory activity, making them especially heart healthy. Research has demonstrated that eating three or more servings of blueberries and strawberries per week may help women reduce their risk of a heart attack by as much as one-third.

Foods highest in anthocyanins include:
- Concord grapes and 100% grape juice made with Concord grapes
- Berries
- Tart cherries and 100% tart cherry juice
- Eggplant
- Red cabbage

though; studies show that obese women following a fruit-enriched low-calorie diet high in antioxidants as opposed to a low-calorie diet alone significantly improve cardiovascular risk factors related to obesity, such as LDL cholesterol. That's proof that it's not just about counting calories; it's about making calories count.

To get the best results, we want to keep our calories balanced as well. There is a reason the portion sizes of fruits and veggies that I recommend are so much larger than the portion sizes I recommend for meats and fats. It's all about increasing your intake of these powerful antioxidants so that you can get all the benefits.

Research shows that combining increased fruit and vegetable intake with decreased fat intake is an effective strategy for managing body weight while controlling hunger. By following the *Schedule Me Skinny* meal pattern and menu plan, you'll get to feel firsthand how antioxidants work in this way.

VITAMIN D AND CALCIUM

Powerhouse nutrients vitamin D and calcium may lead to a beneficial reduction in abdominal fat in overweight and obese adults. Research also found that consumption of calcium and vitamin D during a weight-loss intervention enhanced the beneficial effects of body weight loss on heart health in overweight or obese women with usual low daily calcium intake.

Foods highest in both vitamin D and calcium include:

○ Fortified low-fat dairy products like milk, cheese, and yogurt
○ Salmon, especially salmon canned with bones
○ Fortified cereals

Studies have shown that vitamin D and calcium are beneficial to weight loss. In fact, not getting enough calcium may trigger the release of calcitriol, a hormone that causes the body to store fat. Scientists at the University of Tennessee found that people on a reduced-calorie diet who included an extra 300 to 400 milligrams of calcium a day lost significantly more weight than those who ate the same number of calories but with less calcium. Scientists aren't exactly sure why, but eating calcium-rich foods is more effective than taking calcium supplements, so including these nutrient-rich foods in your diet throughout the day is important.

 ## REAL-LIFE SUCCESS STORY

learned so many things from Sarah-Jane, but the one thing that stands out the most is not to deprive myself. Occasional treats are okay! But she also helped me change my idea of what a treat is (a treat can be a 70-calorie frozen yogurt bar; it doesn't have to be a mammoth bowl of ice cream with chocolate syrup) and how frequently I can enjoy that treat (not more than once a day). Sarah-Jane also encouraged me to look at *why* I wanted a treat and ways that I can "reward" myself without using food, such as taking a walk, reading a magazine, taking time to call an old friend. Sarah-Jane taught me to look at food as fuel rather than something to keep from being bored, or to comfort me when I'm tired, or to calm me down when I'm angry. The only thing food can fix is true, physical hunger. If hunger is not the problem, then food is not the solution. Getting control of my eating helped me feel better about myself in every aspect of my life. It has a ripple effect; when you achieve your weight goals, other things (like deadlines, piles of laundry, stress) seem to become more manageable, too!

—*Mary Lee B.*

TIP FROM MARY LEE: We are all given the same amount of time every day, the same 24 hours to spend however we choose. It is extremely important that you make it a priority to spend time on yourself, so that you can be the healthiest person possible. And once your body is healthier, your brain will function better, your relationships with your children and husband will improve. . . . It does take time to get healthy, but the investment of time for yourself is worth every minute!

If you're getting worried about having the time to stock your kitchen with all these great meal and snack options, never fear! In Chapter 5 I will share with you the secrets to getting in and out of the grocery store fast, all while slashing your grocery bill and leaving with a cart full of these healthy foods!

CHAPTER 5

GET IN, GET OUT, GET GROCERIES THAT WILL GET YOU FIT

Now that you know the Schedule Me Skinny plan that will help you peel the pounds off despite your busy schedule, let's talk about how to get you in and out of the grocery store super fast and with as much cash still in your wallet as possible!

Eating Healthy for Less

Is it possible to get the healthy foods that this meal pattern recommends without breaking the bank? Yes, but how you shop is important. According to the Food Marketing Institute, for every minute we spend in the grocery store, we spend $2! The quicker we

MEAT AND POULTRY TIPS: WHEN POSSIBLE AND AFFORDABLE, OPT FOR . . .

1 **Lean.** Whether it's lean poultry or lean beef, the lean stuff has less artery-clogging saturated fat. The leaner the cut, the better!

2 **"Naturally raised."** A USDA term meaning the animal wasn't given antibiotics, growth hormones, or animal by-products.

3 **No nitrates/nitrites.** These are potentially harmful preservatives sometimes found in cured meats, hot dogs, sausages, and bacon. You'll find them on the ingredients list. Research shows that excessive amounts can have a carcinogenic effect. "Natural" meats don't have these ingredients, but unfortunately the USDA doesn't regulate this approved term.

4 **Wild salmon.** There's no such thing as organic fish, but we do know that choosing wild instead of farmed guarantees far fewer contaminants, less overall fat, and more of the healthy omega-3 fats.

get our groceries, the less money we'll probably spend. And believe it or not, healthy grocery shopping does not require hours of planning and label reading if you have a shopping strategy like this one:

1. Make your list by area of the store. This arrangement of the list will eliminate running back and forth across the store as well as ensure that you don't miss anything. One trip around the store and you are done!

- **Organic.** Though organic meat is ideal, it is by no means necessary for a healthy diet. And it's quite pricey! Hormones are not used in producing organic meats, and pesticides are not used in producing the feed. Buying organic chicken is a surefire way to avoid antibiotics, but there's no need to worry about hormones. Though hormones may be given to cows, hormone use in poultry and pork has been prohibited since 1959! If organic is out of your price range, that's okay, too!

- **Grass-fed meat.** Save this pricey option for a splurge. "Grass-fed" means that the animals are fed on their mother's milk, hay, and grass instead of grains. Some research suggests that grass-fed meat is overall lower in fat while higher in heart-healthy omega-3 fats and antioxidants than meat from grain-fed cattle.

2. Don't get distracted by items that aren't on your list. If you pick up an item, you are four times more likely to buy it than if you don't touch it. Save time and avoid junk-food impulse buys by keeping your hands free of anything that's not on your list.

3. Call ahead. Not sure which grocery store is most likely to have a certain ingredient? Give your usual store a ring and ask if it is something they carry and if so, on which aisle you can find it. The customer service departments are there for these very questions and calling to ask can save you a wasted trip to the store. Plus, it will prevent a time-wasting scavenger hunt to find the item once you arrive.

4. Follow the 80/20 rule. Do 80% of your shopping around the perimeter of the store, where the whole-food groups such as produce, dairy, and lean meats live, and just 20% of your shopping down the aisles, focusing on frozen veggies and whole-grain products like breads, cereals, rice, and pasta. Staying mostly around the perimeter may help to ensure that you stick to the healthy items on your list and avoid wasting time by being tempted by junk food.

Quick Couponing

Clipping coupons to save a dollar here and there is a thing of the past. There are now dozens of paper-free tools to make saving money at the grocery store easier than ever. Take the scissors out of savings with these quick couponing tips!

1. **Food on the Table:** This app makes meal planning a breeze by offering delicious and simple recipes designed to help families eat better and save money along the way. After you enter your family's food preferences, the meal planner uses your phone's GPS to track down the best finds at local stores. You can either print the organized grocery list or view it on your smartphone. The best part is that it features chef-approved recipes that even the kids will love! Say hello to stress-free bargain grocery shopping!
2. **SnipSnap:** Hate forgetting your coupons at home? This app takes the stress out of couponing by offering discount coupons through your phone—no paper needed! Basically, it allows you to scan the paper coupons to create a digital copy and even sends you expiration-date alerts and in-store reminders so you don't forget to use them.
3. **Grocery Smarts:** If you're an extreme couponer, this one

is for you. This clever app helps you save time and money by scanning the weekly flyers for popular stores like Walmart and comparing the prices to find the best deal. Why not shop for what's on sale each week?

4. **Supercook.com:** This fabulous free Web site helps you create delicious recipes with whatever ingredients you have in your pantry. If you've got a package of beef sitting in the fridge and no idea what to do with it, Supercook can help!

5. **Shortcuts.com:** Check out this simple Web site for the lowest prices around on your favorite foods.

6. **Coupons.com:** This Web site has tons of coupons for everything from toothpaste to yogurt. Check it out before you head to the grocery store for a variety of fantastic deals!

Buy Generic, Bulk, and Canned

Store brands (or generics) tend to be the same quality as name-brand food items with a price tag that is already 20% cheaper. To save even more, use coupons to stock up on store brands at the end of the month, as that is when store brands typically go on sale (in contrast to name-brand items, which tend to go on sale at the beginning of the month, when most people are paid).

Buy in bulk, but only for items that you use regularly. Buying in bulk at warehouse stores can save you money, as they often offer a

WHAT'S ORGANIC?

To be designated as "organic," items must be produced without genetic engineering, hormones, or antibiotics. The USDA organic seal means that the product is at least 95% organic. You may also see "100% organic" labels, meaning that 100% of the ingredients are organic. Last, the label "made with organic ingredients" means that at least 70% of the ingredients are organic. Organic produce and meats tend to be pricier, but if exposure to pesticides and antibiotics is a concern for you, organic may be the way to go. A cheaper option may be the "naturally raised" label, which denotes that the animal wasn't given any antibiotics, growth hormones, or animal by-products.

QUINOA 101

Did you know that the Food and Agricultural Organization of the United Nations (FAO) officially declared the year 2013 the "International Year of Quinoa"? Here's your guide on how to select it, store it, and cook it for perfectly fluffy quinoa every time:

How to select it: Quinoa comes in a variety of colors, from off-white and red to black. They all taste and cost pretty much the same, except organic varieties, which are a bit more costly. It can be found prepackaged or in the bulk section of natural health-food stores and regular supermarkets as well.

How to store it: Quinoa should be stored in an airtight container. If you won't be using it for a while, store it in the fridge for 3–6 months.

How to cook it: Quinoa has a natural bitter outer coating of saponins, so you'll want to rinse it with cold water in a fine-mesh sieve right before cooking. Some varieties come pre-rinsed, so make sure to read the label. To cook it, place one part quinoa in a pot with two parts liquid, like water, or vegetable broth for extra flavor. Bring the mixture to a boil, then reduce the heat to low and simmer, covered, for about 15 minutes, or until all the liquid is absorbed. The quinoa will double in size, and you'll notice a bunch of white-spiraled tails—that's normal. Fluff with a fork and serve. For a nuttier flavor, dry-roast it in a skillet over medium-low heat for five minutes, stirring constantly, before cooking.

quantity discount, but even if it looks like a great price, if it is a food item that you don't use regularly, it may go bad before you have the chance to use it. To make fresh foods that you buy in bulk last longer, keep them in the freezer (check out some of these items on the Freezer Must-Haves list in Chapter 4).

The meal pattern calls for lots of servings of colorful fruits and veggies. To save on these filling, healthy foods, you can use canned or frozen fruits and vegetables instead of fresh produce. They will keep longer and often have the same nutritional value as fresh foods. Just be sure to rinse and drain canned veggies to reduce the sodium by 40%. And check the ingredients list for canned or frozen fruits to make sure that they have no added sugar.

10 MUST-HAVES FOR $2 OR LESS

1 Frozen veggies, $2/package
2 Canned beans (black or garbanzo), 89 cents
3 16-oz. box whole-grain spaghetti, $1.31
4 6 oz. canned wild salmon, $1.79
5 1 lb. California grapes, $1.99
6 3 lbs. bananas, $1.77
7 6 eggs, $1.09
8 ½ gallon skim milk, $2
9 9-oz. bag fresh spinach, $2
10 8 oz. nonfat Greek yogurt, 89 cents

Eat Local to Eat for Less

One easy way to get the most nutritional bang for your buck is to buy your food locally. Shopping at farmers' markets or choosing food at the grocery store that is labeled as locally grown means that you are getting the freshest items possible, since they haven't had to travel thousands of miles to get to you. And fresher food, especially fresh produce, tends to be more nutritious food, since it hasn't had time to lose nutrients along the way.

Plus, locally grown food just tastes better. Maybe this is because it is fresher or maybe it is simply because you will be consuming it right at the season's peak. Either way, I will take a juicy red tomato straight from a farmer over a transported, store-bought one any day.

Not to mention it gives me such peace of mind to know where my food is coming from. It is so cool to meet the farmer who grew the veggies I'll be eating and ask him questions. If you don't have time for a leisurely trip to the farmers' market, never fear! You can get all these benefits and more by joining a CSA (see breakout box). Farmers often deliver CSA baskets straight to their members' neighborhoods or offices. That's like someone doing your healthy grocery shopping for you—and you get the freshest, most flavorful items available! Score!

Quick Dinners on the Fly

If all the food prep you want to do is picking up takeout on the way home from work, try heading to your grocery store instead. You'll be able to find a prepared healthy meal that's fresher than the drive-through offerings and just as fast. If you are a fish fan, head to the seafood counter and ask them to steam some shrimp for you. Most grocery stores will provide this service free of charge, and the great thing is not only can you get just the amount of shrimp you need, but you can also choose your seasoning! Pair the steamed shrimp with some microwavable brown rice and veggies, and you have a balanced meal in minutes.

Rotisserie chicken is also an easy grab-and-go grocery store dinner option. It will provide lean protein for several meals (just pull off the skin to keep the calorie count in check), and you can add it to different dishes to keep things interesting. Try it on top of a salad, in a wrap, or tossed with whole-grain pasta and veggies.

Almost every grocery store these days has a sushi station. Choose a brown rice roll (avoid anything tempura-style, since that means it has been fried) and pair it with some Asian-style microwavable veggies for a super-simple supper.

So, what if you want to make your own dinner with all this great healthy local food that you got on the cheap? In the next chapter, I'll

EAT LOCALLY WITH A CSA

Have you heard about CSAs? That's community-supported agriculture. CSAs have become a great and popular way for people to buy local and seasonal foods directly from a farmer. The idea is simple:

1 A farmer offers a certain number of "shares" to the public.
2 The share is a box of vegetables and other farm products.
3 Interested consumers purchase a share for a season (usually from $400 to $700) and in return receive a box of seasonal produce each week throughout the farming season.

Sound interesting? Check out all the advantages this arrangement creates:

Advantages for Farmers

- Get to spend time marketing the food early in the year.
- Receive payment early in the season, which helps with the farm's cash flow.
- Have an opportunity to get to know the people who eat the food they grow.

Advantages for Consumers

- Eat fresh food, with all the flavor and nutritional benefits.
- Get exposed to new fruits and vegetables that are in season.
- Develop a relationship with the farmer who grows their food and learn more about how food is grown.

It's a simple enough idea, but its impact has been profound. Want to find a CSA in your area? Visit http://www.localharvest.org/csa/.

show you how to cook it up in minutes. In the same amount of time that it will take you to sit in the drive-through line, you can prepare a quick, healthy, and delicious meal! You just have to know how! In Chapter 6, I dish on the basic cooking skills, kitchen tools, and cooking shortcuts that you need to know to maximize the time you spend in the kitchen.

KICKIN' IT IN THE KITCHEN, *SKINNY* STYLE

Let me get real with you about something. You don't have to cook *at all* in order to lose weight—you really don't. You could eat weight-loss bars and shakes, or frozen meals, until you can't stand to even look at them anymore, and you might achieve some weight loss. But if you want that weight loss to be lasting, and if you want to develop healthy habits that make maintenance a breeze, plus reap the benefits of nourishing food, you'll need to be able to cook—at least a little bit.

The good news is that I am not talking spending hours slaving away over the stove. I'm talking basic skills that will allow you to throw together a healthy meal using real food in just minutes on busy weeknights. If you are a cooking diva, you may already know these basic culinary skills, but no judgment if you are not. Below, I give you the step-by-step how-to on everything you wanted to know about basic cooking for weight loss but were afraid to ask!

I. HOW TO BOIL EGGS

➢ Place eggs in a pot filled with **cold water**. Water should cover eggs by 1 to 2 inches.

➢ **Boil the water.** Bring water to a full boil and cover the pot. Turn off the heat, remove the pot from the burner, and let it stand, covered, for 12 minutes.

➢ **Submerge the eggs in cold water.** Drain the pot and transfer the eggs to a bowl of cold water.

➢ **Crack and peel the eggs.** Tap each egg a few times to crack its shell, then roll it on a work surface to break the shell completely. Start peeling, dunking the egg into the bowl of water as you go to wash away any bits of shell.

2. HOW TO CHOP, MINCE, AND DICE VEGETABLES

These techniques may vary depending on the vegetable, but they use the same basics.

➢ **Chop.** Grasp a chef's knife with one hand and rest the other hand on the top front of the knife for control. Chop in large, uniform pieces, using quick, heavy rocking motions.

➢ **Mince.** You'll often see this word on recipes that call for garlic or shallots. It means to cut the food into tiny pieces that don't have to be perfectly uniform in size. To achieve a mince, simply slice the food into several smaller pieces. Then stack the pieces side by side and place your knife in a horizontal position over the pieces. Then rock your knife back and forth across the pieces while maintaining contact with the cutting board. Place the hand that is not holding the knife on the spine of the knife to guide it as you mince. Just be sure to keep your fingers up and out of the way of the blade!

➢ **Dice.** Cut the vegetable lengthwise into even slices, then stack the slices and cut them into long sticks. Gather the sticks and cut them crosswise into cubes. Make sure to get the cubes as even as you can.

3. HOW TO ROAST POULTRY (CHICKEN AND TURKEY)

➤ **Preheat the oven** to 375°F for chicken and 325°F–350°F for turkey.

➤ **Rinse** the whole bird thoroughly. Pat dry with paper towels. Make sure the giblets have been removed.

➤ **Place bird, breast side up, on an oven rack in a shallow roasting pan.** Brush with cooking oil and, if desired, sprinkle with a crushed dried herb, such as thyme or oregano.

➤ **Cover bird with foil,** leaving air space between bird and foil. Lightly press the foil to the ends of the drumsticks and neck to enclose bird.

➤ **Roast.** Depending on the size, a chicken should roast for 1–2½ hours and a turkey should roast 2½–5 hours (research specific roasting time by weight online). Two-thirds of the way through the roasting time, cut band of skin between drumsticks. Uncover bird for the last 45 minutes of roasting for larger birds or the last 30 minutes of roasting for smaller birds.

➤ **Continue roasting** until internal temperature of the bird reaches 165°F (use a meat thermometer and make sure it's not touching the bone) and when the juices run clear upon puncturing with a fork.

➤ **Remove bird from oven.** Cover. Allow it to rest for 15 minutes before carving.

4. HOW TO COOK AND BROWN LEAN GROUND BEEF

➤ **Heat a nonstick skillet or an iron skillet and add the beef.** Warm the pan over medium to medium-high heat. Add beef to the center of the pan.

> **Break the meat into large pieces.** Use a stiff spatula to break the ground meat into several pieces.

> **Break the meat into smaller pieces and brown.** Continue breaking the ground meat into smaller and smaller pieces. Sprinkle with salt and any spices you are using. Stir the beef occasionally to make sure it's browning evenly.

> **Finish browning.** The beef has finished when it is evenly browned and shows no signs of pink. Break open a few of the larger crumbles to be sure that it has browned all the way through.

5. HOW TO SAUTÉ VEGETABLES

This is an easy way to give vegetables flavor and texture, while still cooking them all the way through.

> **Wash, dry, and cut up vegetables.**

> **Heat** a small amount (1 teaspoon per serving of veggies) of olive oil in a large, shallow pan on the stove over medium to high heat.

> **Add the vegetables to the hot pan.**

> **Stir the vegetables frequently until they're nicely browned and cooked through.** Stir the vegetables every so often with a wooden spoon or spatula. If it looks like the vegetables are getting too brown, but aren't cooked through yet, turn the heat down a bit.

6. HOW TO BAKE A POTATO (IN THE MICROWAVE!)

Who said this had to be done in an oven? This is a fast, easy way to bake a potato.

> **Wash and dry the potato.**

> **Using a fork, poke holes in the potato to vent steam.** Aim to get 3 or 4 pokes on each area: top, bottom, and 2 sides. Or you can cut a deep "X" into the long side with a knife.

> **Wrap the potato in a wet paper towel and put it on a plate.**

COOKING SECRETS FROM SEASONED CHEFS

I asked some of the culinary geniuses and professional chefs in my life to share their favorite secrets for making cooking easier and more fun. Use their tips to make your time in the kitchen a breeze!

1. **Put a head of garlic in the microwave for 20 seconds** to make peeling the cloves a breeze! And if your hands smell garlicky afterward, rub them on your stainless-steel sink and then wash them to take the smell away.

2. **Cover a pot of water with the lid to help it boil faster.**

3. **Before you start cooking, gather all your ingredients and put them in one place.** Chefs actually have a name for this: "mise en place," which is French for "putting in place." This will save you time and make cooking less stressful.

4. **Before you start cooking, give the whole recipe a quick read.** This will take just a couple of minutes, but it will prevent you from making a time-costing mistake like forgetting to preheat the oven or to chop an onion.

5. **If you are grilling or pan-searing meat or fish, don't flip it too much.** Put it on the heat and then leave it there for the recommended cook time per side. Then, and only then, try to flip it. If it comes right up, it is ready to be flipped. This will also help you avoid having food stuck to the pan that will take lots of time and elbow grease to scrub off.

(Continued)

6 **If you want veggies to cook faster, cut them into smaller pieces.** Just be sure that your pieces are also uniform to avoid having some pieces cook faster than others.

7 **If you're not sure how to cook a veggie, chop it, toss with a little olive oil, salt, and pepper, and roast at a high heat (around 400°F) until tender.** This method makes pretty much any veggie taste amazing.

8 If you want the lovely flavor of a pan-seared meat but don't want to waste time standing at the stove to cook it, **sear just the outside of each side of the meat** and then finish by baking it in the oven.

➤ **Put the plate in the microwave and cook.** Use 3 minutes for a very small potato, 4½ minutes for a medium-sized, 6 minutes for a large, and 7 to 8 minutes for a huge potato. Increase the times by about two-thirds for multiple potatoes (for instance, 2 large potatoes would be 10 minutes).

➤ **Let the potato rest for 5 minutes.** This allows the core of the potato to finish cooking with the heat that is trapped in the inner layers. Wrapping it in aluminum foil after taking it out of the microwave will help speed this process.

➤ **Cut open the potato, garnish it with toppings of your choice, and enjoy!** For a complete meal, try topping it with chili and veggies.

Of course, in addition to knowing these basic skills, you can always follow a recipe. There really is some truth to the saying that if you can read, you can cook. Most recipes assume just a very basic knowledge of cooking and culinary terms and will walk you through the preparation of the dish with very clear, step-by-step instructions.

It is not just what you put into the dish, but how you cook it that can play a large role in taste! Poaching and pan-frying, for example, do an excellent job of locking in and bringing out flavors of food, without adding all the fat that comes with methods such as deep frying. Check out these cooking methods to add some flavor without the calories!

In addition to familiar grilling, roasting, and baking, these are among the healthiest cooking methods you'll see in recipes:

- ➤ **Blanching:** Blanching is a technique in which a food is submerged in boiling water for a brief time and then plunged into ice water to stop the cooking process. This process not only gives fresh veggies a beautiful, bright color, but it's also super quick. And a quick cooking time means nutrients and that great crunchy texture are both preserved.
- ➤ **Poaching:** To poach a food means to simmer it in a liquid other than oil—usually wine, stock, or milk. The best thing about poaching foods is that you don't have to use added fat, and yet your dish won't end up dry. Eggs are popular candidates for poaching, but fish and poultry are great poached as well.
- ➤ **Pan Frying:** Pan frying is to fry something using minimal oil

or fat. If you like fried foods, but you don't want to sabotage your weight loss, this is a go-to cooking method for you. You need just enough oil in your pan so that the food doesn't stick, and if you have a nonstick pan or iron skillet, you can get by with a light mist of cooking oil spray. Pan frying is a tasty and fast way to cook up a healthy fish dish.

Adding Flavor the Healthy Way

Now that you know how to cook a healthy dish, let's talk about adding some healthy flavor! Adding flavor doesn't mean going wild with the saltshaker or tossing tons of butter and saturated fat into your dish. There are countless seasonings, ingredients, and cooking methods that can amp up the flavor without putting a damper on nutrition.

Herbs and spices are crucial for adding the finishing touches to a dish. Refer to the "Top 10 Herbs and Spices for the Busy Cook" breakout box to know which spices and herbs go well with different dishes! Low-sodium options of spice blends are now available to add zest to your meal without the bloat-inducing sodium overload. Mrs. Dash is a great line of low-sodium spice blends. They make a variety of blends for almost every kind of dish, from Southwestern-style fare to Italian eats. So skip the saltshaker and spice it up! Try the Mrs. Dash Southwest Chipotle Seasoning in the **Pulled Pork Tacos** slow-cooker recipe.

There are a few go-to ingredients to call on when it comes to amping up flavor. Take leeks, for example. They can be substituted for onions to add a slightly sweeter flavor to salads, soups, and side dishes. Chives are another flavor favorite. Top off your veggies or fish with fresh chives to add zip without the harshness that an onion sometimes brings.

An easy way to skip the salt is to add citrus instead. Lemons and limes squeezed or zested over vegetables, fish, or meat can perk up the dish, while keeping it light in sodium. Or if you are bored with plain water, use some citrus slices (try a variety of lemons, limes, and oranges) to add flavor while keeping it calorie-free. Try lemons in the **No-Mess Baked Fish and Veggies** recipe.

Nothing can add healthy flavor quite like salsa. Salsa brings tons of flavor and very few calories! It is great to throw in with eggs, vegetables, or even to top off some meat or fish dishes. Try salsa in the **Black Jack Tacos** or **Lentil Stuffed Peppers** recipes.

Cooking a South American dish? Add some minced hot peppers and BAM! Your dish is taken to the next level. Just be sure to remove the seeds first if you don't like things too spicy! Another easy way to add a flavorful kick to any dish is to add freshly ground black pepper. As an added bonus, research shows that pepperine, a compound found in pepper, may help to reduce the activity of genes that form fat cells!

Flavored vinegars are another must-have to add flavor when cooking slimming meals. Vinegars can be added to sauces, dressing, soups, and really anything else your heart desires! There are countless flavored vinegars to choose from; my personal favorite is balsamic vinegar. Make your own salad dressing by combining two parts healthy oil (like olive oil or canola oil) with one part of your favorite vinegar, along with salt, pepper, and herbs to taste. Whisk together and the dressing is ready to drizzle on your greens!

Finally, my favorite flavor superstar is the sun-dried tomato. If I'm cooking anything Italian, you can bet that I am throwing in some sun-dried tomatoes to finish off the dish. These tomatoes are flavor packed, nutrient dense, and delicious. Taste their perfection in the **Pasta with Sautéed Spinach, Toasted Pine Nuts, and Chicken** "Plan B" recipe.

TOP 10 HERBS AND SPICES FOR THE BUSY COOK

Herb or Spice	Flavor	Dishes
Cinnamon	Warm and bitter-sweet	Sprinkle on oatmeal, vanilla yogurt, or apples. Put a pinch in coffee or tea. Try in Indian and Moroccan dishes to add flavor to meats, stews, soups, and curries.
Dill	Fresh, slight citrus flavor	Use to season fish. Use fresh in salads or dried to season potato dishes.
Rosemary	Floral and evergreen flavor	Use in Italian-style dishes like pasta or bruschetta. Use to season meats and chicken. Use to season roasted potatoes and other veggies.
Nutmeg	Delicate and warm	Use for many baked goods such as cookies or pumpkin dishes. Add to winter squash and spinach dishes. Sprinkle with cinnamon and honey on a sweet potato. Place a pinch in your coffee or tea.
Cumin	Warm, earthy flavor	Use in Southwestern-style dishes. Use to season salsas and guacamole. Use as a rub on grilled meats and poultry.
Garlic Powder	Sharp and pungent, but mellows through the cooking process	Sprinkle into marinara sauce or on roasted vegetables. Sprinkle on chicken, fish, or beef. Add to hummus for enhanced flavor. Sprinkle into vegetable sautés. Add to soups or sauces.
Oregano	Robust and pungent	Sprinkle into marinara sauce. Add to a salad for a Greek flavor. Sprinkle into an omelet with vegetables.

		Combine in seasoning rub for beef, pork, or lamb. Mix with lemon juice and drizzle on fish or chicken. Sauté vegetables with oregano, olive oil, and garlic powder.
Basil	Sweet with a refreshing earthiness	Use to add flavor to Italian and Greek dishes. Improves the flavor of chicken, eggs, fish, beef, and cheese. Add to a tomato salad. Add to pasta dishes or marinara sauce to enhance flavor.
Chili Powder	Fiery and pungent (may be mild or hot depending on peppers it is made from)	Use for Mexican and Southwestern dishes. Add to chili, soups, or stews. Enhance the flavor of fish, chicken, pork, beef, and beans. Add to sautéed vegetables, fajita blends, or tacos.
Thyme	Minty, warm, and peppery	Use for Mediterranean, Cajun, and Creole dishes. Enhance the flavor of chicken, fish, lamb, and eggs. Add to soups, stews, and sauces. Sauté with onions, mushrooms, potatoes, and carrots.

Efficiency in the Kitchen

Not only can being efficient in the kitchen cut down the time you spend chopping and prepping, but it also saves money and allows you to spend more time doing what you love outside of the kitchen! Cooking can be enjoyable, relaxing, and even therapeutic, but if you're just getting home from work and want to get dinner on the table in a flash, efficiency becomes critical. These time-saving tips may just save dinner!

First things first. Read through the recipe and gather all ingredients before you begin to cook so you aren't running back to your cupboard for a bay leaf halfway through the recipe when your hands are covered in sauce. Gather measuring cups, knives, pots, cutting boards, and ingredients and lay them out on your counter in the order that you are going to use them, according to the recipe. Also, take a look at the recipe and make sure your ingredients are properly prepped. Chop everything that needs to be chopped at once, rather than trying to chop each item as you go. Not only will prepping your ingredients first save you time; it will also prevent you from missing an important step in the recipe or burning something in the pan because you didn't have the next ingredient ready at the right time.

Speaking of gathering your ingredients, organizing your kitchen consistently can save you loads of time. Have a specific spot for each type of food and keep it there at all times. For example, always keep cheeses in one drawer of the fridge, veggies in another, meats on the bottom shelf, and yogurts and milk on the top shelf. Then you won't be wasting time on a scavenger hunt for each ingredient. Store dry goods like spices or canned foods in alphabetical order in your pantry so you can spot the one you're looking for in just seconds. Keep items that you use in nearly every recipe, like olive oil or salt and pepper, out on the counter beside the stove for extra-easy access. You can also take this approach with utensils that you use regularly, keeping them within easy reach in a container that stays on the counter.

The most important thing to remember when it comes to efficiency in the kitchen is multitasking. Why chop carrots, sauté onions, then boil water when you can do all three at once? Whenever a recipe calls for an ingredient that needs to be boiled (like pasta), always start by boiling the water with a pinch of salt, since it'll take about 10 minutes for the water to come to a boil. That way, you can chop your veggies while the water is heating up. Same with preheating your oven; it'll take some time to get hot, so check to see if the recipe calls for cooking in the oven, and if it does, preheat the oven, and prep the ingredients while it's getting hot.

Use timers to multitask effectively. Of course you can set a timer to cook something for the appropriate amount of time, but timers can also be useful to remind you about a meat that is marinating or something in the oven that needs to be flipped halfway through. Timers keep your multitasking on track because they help you to remember one task as you are working on another one. If the only timer you have in your kitchen is the one on your oven, consider buying a cheap minute timer or using one on your phone so that you can keep track of the timing of two or more items at once.

Speaking of timing, make sure your recipes don't require that your meat and potatoes and veggies all be cooking in the oven at different temperatures at the same time, unless you are lucky enough to have a kitchen with multiple ovens. Instead, as you plan your meals, choose to combine recipes that have different cooking methods. For example, you might grill your chicken, roast your sweet potatoes in the oven, and sauté your green beans on the top of the stove. That way, everything is done at once and you don't have to wait for one item to finish cooking before you start cooking the next one.

Another way to make sure everything is ready at the same time is to take a close look at all the recipes. Read through all the steps to get a feel for the total time it will take for you to prepare a meal and start with the item that will take the longest.

I wouldn't recommend trying to make more than two or three recipes per meal, and even fewer for beginners. That's because when you are following a recipe (unless you have it memorized) you have to concentrate on it closely and read steps multiple times to make sure you are preparing it correctly. It's setting yourself up for disaster if you try to take on more than two or three recipes at a time. Instead, pick a recipe for your main course and for one side item, and then round out your meal with sides that don't require a recipe, like microwavable whole-grain brown rice, a bagged salad, or sliced fruit. Similarly, I would never try more than one new recipe at once. The first time you make a recipe, it will take the most time because you are not familiar with it. So if you are going to make multiple recipes, be sure that only one is new to you and the others are old favorites; this strategy will keep your efficiency up and your stress level down.

Take shortcuts with the ingredients that often have the most prep work. When it comes to chopped veggies, don't be afraid to go with frozen. Most are frozen at the peak of freshness, so you won't be sacrificing much in flavor and quality. Plus, you can buy inexpensive blends of veggies that are perfect for whatever cuisine you're prepping, like a stir-fry blend with already-chopped mushrooms, peppers, and baby corn or a California blend with zucchini, onions, and broccoli. Or if you're choosing fresh produce, look for the preprepped section, where you can often find chopped onion, chopped celery, peeled and chopped sweet potatoes, prepared salads, and more. Or scoot over to the deli/salad bar section and grab just the amount you need of specific ingredients like hummus, tomato slices, or beans rather than buying a huge container.

Cooking in large batches is another great way to cut down on time and money spent on cooking in the near future. Multiply your meals by making double the amount of stuffed peppers or quinoa casserole, and dinner next week is all ready to go. Simply place leftovers in freezer-safe baggies or Tupperware and label food with the name of the recipe and the date. Labeling is an important time-saver in and of itself, as later on you won't have to open every baggie or container trying to find the leftovers you are looking for.

Keep your kitchen tools useful. Knives need to be sharpened once every couple of weeks to stay safe and effective for chopping and slicing. Using a dull knife can result in an injury or can slow your prep time down.

Think twice before you use an appliance. Is there really any need to use a mixer to beat an egg when a simple whisk will do the job? Do you really need a food processor to turn crackers into crumbs or could you just use the back of a spoon to crush them in their plastic packaging? Should you warm the sauce over the stove or can you just heat it in the microwave? Not only does it often take a long time to get these tools out and set up for use, but you also may be getting additional dishes dirty when there is no need to. That is why it is important to read each step of a recipe and choose the best kitchen tool to complete the task before you get started.

Another way to cut down on cleanup time is to line your pans when you are cooking in the oven. Use either aluminum foil or a silicon mat to cover your pan before placing food in it for cooking. When you are done cooking, your pan is still clean and nothing sticks to it!

Ice cube trays aren't just for ice! After all, who uses a whole can of tomato paste? Use the perfectly portioned spaces to store extra pesto, veggie purees to add to sauces, tomato paste, and fresh herbs frozen with a bit of water. Pop out a cube anytime you need a small portion, so they don't go to waste and you won't have to measure out the amount you need each time (each cube is about a tablespoon and they can be used directly from frozen).

Last, try to clean little by little as you go. Pull a Rachael Ray and keep a scrap bowl out so you don't end up with onion peels and pepper seeds all over the counter. You'll keep your cooking area clean, giving you more space to work without wasting time on multiple trips to the trash can. You can just toss all your scraps in the bowl and then empty it once you are totally finished cooking.

Instead of creating a stressful mound of dishes in the sink, rinse dirty dishes right away and put them in the dishwasher. This will prevent wasted time scrubbing off junk that will cake on the pans if they are allowed to sit unrinsed. Whenever you're finished with the milk or the cinnamon, put it back in the fridge or the spice cabinet.

Change your clothes. You may be eager to get dinner on the table as soon as you get home from work, but you're not going to be very efficient if you're trying to keep your hair out of your face or your suit clean. Not to mention that peep toe heels aren't exactly safe or comfortable to wear while cooking. So put your hair in a ponytail, put on comfortable clothing, and change into your tennies to get serious in the kitchen. An added bonus of this attire is that you can also do some of the multitasking exercises that you'll find in Chapter 8 while you wait for dinner to cook. Now that's efficiency!

Keeping Your Food Safe

1. **Be Smart When You Heat and Eat.** In your haste to cook a healthy meal quickly, don't forget it's important to cook your food safely too, which means making sure it heats to the correct internal temperature. The "Is it done?" question can be enough to stress out any cook. I recommend using a digital meat thermometer to quickly determine if your dish is ready to eat. It's ready when it reaches the temperatures outlined in the chart below:

ITEM	TEMPS
Refrigerator	Keep below 40°F
Freezer	Keep below 0°F
Leftovers	Heat to at least 165°F
Poultry	Heat to 165°F
Beef and Pork	Heat to 160°F
Fish	Heat to 145°F
Egg Dishes	Heat to 160°F

2. **Know When to Toss It.** A busy schedule can lend itself to a bad memory sometimes, and it can even make you sick if

HOW TO PROPERLY FREEZE FOODS

The freezer is a great tool for both keeping food safe to eat and having easy, healthy food options on hand anytime. Here are some tips so you can freeze with ease.

- **Choose freezer-friendly foods.** Some foods are better suited to freezing and reheating than others. Casseroles, soups, stews, chili, and meat loaf all stand up to the freezer well.
- **Chill.** To keep food safe, cool freshly cooked dishes quickly before freezing. Place food in a shallow, wide container and refrigerate, uncovered, until cool. To chill soup or stew even faster, pour it into a metal bowl and set it in an ice bath.
- **Store.** Avoid freezer burn by using moisture-proof zip-top plastic bags and wrap. Remove the air from bags before sealing. Store soups and stews in freezer bags, which can be placed flat and freeze quickly. Store foods in small servings, no more than I quart, to help them freeze quickly. Use a permanent marker to label each container with the name of the dish, volume or weight if you've measured it, and the date you put it in the freezer.
- **Freeze quickly.** Do not crowd the freezer—arrange containers in a single layer to allow enough room for air to circulate around them so food will freeze rapidly. Most cooked dishes will keep for 2–3 months in the freezer.
- **When ready to eat, defrost.** Defrost food in the refrigerator or in the microwave. It's best to allow enough time for the food to defrost in the refrigerator—roughly 5 hours per pound. To avoid the risk of contamination, never defrost food at room temperature.

it means accidentally eating food that is too old. However, you don't want to unnecessarily toss healthy food, wasting money when you do, either. So here's a guide on how long you can keep foods and when they have seen their better days. To make things even easier and more accurate, keep a permanent marker and some sticky notes by the fridge and mark foods with the date when you put them away.

ITEM	FREEZE/COOK WITHIN ...	STORE IN FREEZER FOR ...
Raw ground meat, poultry, fish	1–2 days	Max of 4 months
Fresh meat cuts	3–5 days	Max of 4–12 months
Fresh poultry cuts	3–5 days	Max of 9 months
Cooked meat and poultry	3–4 days	Max of 2–3 months
Cooked meals or restaurant meals (Leftovers)	3–4 days	Max of 2–3 months

Kitchen Essentials

Quick cooking can easily become a reality for you if you have the right tools to do it. While you may not be a world-class chef, hopefully you already have some of the basic cooking tools on hand. In addition to a baking sheet, two cutting boards (one for meat and one for produce), measuring cups and spoons, a spatula, mixing spoon, wooden spoon, whisk, citrus squeezer, can opener, and at least one large and one small pan/pot, I suggest checking out these handy kitchen appliances and accessories to make your life easier and your cooking faster!

TOP 10 KITCHEN ESSENTIALS

1. HAND BLENDER

➤ Make smoothies in the included container for on-the-go snacks.

➤ Make soups with your own fresh and healthy ingredients.

➤ Make your own healthy dips and salsas.

➤ Use in place of a food processor for fast chopping.

Added Bonus: This blender takes up very little space, is less expensive than most blenders and mixers, but has both capabilities.

MY PREFERRED: *KitchenAid 3-Speed Hand Blender, $79.99*

2. OIL SPRITZER

➤ Spray oil on salads to control amount of oil.

➤ Spray veggies you plan to roast instead of tossing in oil, which is messier, takes more time, and can cause veggies to be soggy and higher in calories.

➤ Use in place of cooking spray for an additive-free option.

MY PREFERRED: *Misto Olive Oil Sprayer, $10.00*

3. COOKING MAT

➤ Place on baking sheet for roasting veggies, baking cookies, etc. Allows for less butter or oil.

➤ Go green! You no longer have to toss parchment paper or aluminum foil every time you cook.

➤ Reduce cleanup time! You won't have to wash your pan after it has been lined with the cooking mat. Simply rinse the mat in hot water, and you're good to go!

MY PREFERRED: *Silpat mat 8.25" x 11.75", $15.99*

4. LUNCH BOX KITS

➤ Pack your lunch the night before and snap in the ice inserts in the morning. Even if you don't have a fridge at work, you can put these containers in a cooler and be ready!

➤ Pack anything. There are a lot of size options: sandwich, salad, sides, dressings, etc.

MY PREFERRED: *Rubbermaid Lunchblox entree kit $16.99*

5. PROGRAMMABLE SLOW-COOKER

➤ Cook virtually any meal: oatmeal for breakfast, soups, stews, casseroles, etc., for lunch or dinner. Makes enough for the whole family and/or leftovers, which can be frozen for later.

➤ Have meals ready when you are. The small amount of prep that most slow-cooker recipes call for, combined with the programmable feature, allows you to have a delicious, healthy hot meal ready anytime, on even the busiest of days.

MY PREFERRED: *Crock-Pot Programmable Crock-Pot: $39.99*

6. COLLAPSIBLE SALAD SPINNER

➤ Wash and dry salad greens or other fruits and veggies, and since it comes with a removable strainer, you can even use it to drain pasta or rinse and drain canned beans to reduce their sodium content.

➤ Pull the strainer out and use the main bowl to serve the salad or pasta for less cleanup.

MY PREFERRED: *Progressive International Collapsible Salad Spinner: $22.99*

7. MIXING BOWL SET

➤ Reduce dishwashing. You can prep food and serve in these containers if the recipe allows. They also have lids, which means food can be prepped in advance and stored in the fridge, or leftovers can stay in the container and be put back in the fridge.

➤ Warm up leftovers, since they are also microwavable and dishwasher-safe!

MY PREFERRED: *Pyrex Smart Essentials Mixing Bowl Set (8 pieces): $20.69*

PICKING THE BEST SLOW-COOKER

After a long day at work, there's nothing better than coming home to a home-cooked meal ready and waiting for you. Sound too good to be true? Not if you've got a slow-cooker!

If you're in the market for a slow-cooker, keep these features in mind:

Must-Haves

- Removable interior bowl for easy cleaning.
- Glass lid for easy cleaning and durability. Glass lids are likely to last longer than a lid with a metal rim or plastic handles.

Handy Helpers

- Programmable/delayed start
- High, medium, low and keep-warm temperature settings
- Digital temperature display
- Attached thermometer
- Removable cord

Now that you know all about buying a slow-cooker, you'll want to get cooking. Here's what you need to know about using your slow-cooker.

Cooking Tips

- To make cleanup really easy, line the slow-cooker with a cooking bag.
- Make sure all the meat is defrosted before putting it in the slow-cooker so that it will reach a safe food temperature quickly and cook evenly.
- If you need to alter cooking times, keep in mind that 1 hour on the high setting is equal to 2 hours on the low temperature setting.

8. QUALITY KNIFE SET

Good knives are essential for healthy cooking, as they allow you to do everything from chopping, slicing, and dicing fresh fruits and veggies to mincing fresh garlic and herbs to diving into a juicy, lean steak. Plus, knives that are not sharp and high in quality can be dangerous, since old, dull knives actually lead to more skin cuts than sharp ones do.

- Slice fresh bread, chop, slice or dice fresh produce, cut up meat, and more!
- Use the kitchen shears to open packaging and to chop fresh herbs the easy and quick way!

MY PREFERRED: *Calphalon 18-Piece Knife Set: $149.95*

9. IRON SKILLET

- Make fajitas on the grill, simmer spaghetti sauce on the stove, cook a chicken dish in the oven, and more!
- Use on any cooking surface (except in the microwave).
- Add flavor and the important nutrient, iron, to all the food you cook in the skillet.
- Use in place of nonstick or other cookware.
- Quick to clean—just rinse well with hot water and wipe dry with a towel.

MY PREFERRED: *Lodge 10¼-inch Seasoned Skillet, $24.95*

10. SMALL INDOOR GRILL

- Grill foods with ease—fresh or frozen.
- A nonstick, dishwasher-safe surface allows for quick cleanup.
- An easy and healthy way to cook fish, chicken, beef, pork, or veggies in just minutes!

MY PREFERRED: *George Foreman 2-Serving Classic Plate Grill: $19.99*

If something you are cooking doesn't turn out perfectly the first time, don't be discouraged. Anyone can learn to cook, but it can take a little time to feel totally comfortable in the kitchen. I love to cook now, but it wasn't always that way.

When I was in college, my roommates loved cooking and sharing recipes, but I couldn't believe cooking was something people actually enjoyed. The extent of my cooking was heating up a frozen meal or making a sandwich.

But when I met my husband, all that changed. He had mentioned that his mom was a great cook, and you know what they say about a man's stomach and his heart. So for the first time I had a reason to cook and someone to cook for. Now I cook even when my husband is away because I have realized that I am worth cooking for as well.

During one of my first adventures in the kitchen, I almost burned down a whole apartment building. My husband and I were dating at the time, and I wanted to make him a delicious meal for his birthday. Shrimp was going to be the main course, and so I heated a pan on high filled with plenty of oil (big mistake!). I got the shrimp out of the fridge, and when I turned back around, the pan was bursting with flames. We tried throwing water on it (another big mistake— grease fires have to be suffocated by covering them; water just makes it worse), but the flames were already licking the cabinets by that time. Thankfully, the firefighters got there quickly and put the flames out before too much damage was done. We ended up ordering pizza for dinner.

That just goes to show that sometimes things don't turn out, and that everyone needs a Plan B sometimes. So read on. In Chapter 7, I'll tell you what to do on those nights when Plan B means going out to grab a bite.

GIRLS' NIGHT OUT

Getting out and having a good time is key to leading a fun, balanced, and, yes, even healthy life. If anyone ever asked me to give up my social life in order to lose weight, I wouldn't do it. And you shouldn't either. Being healthy involves not just physical health but emotional and spiritual health as well. Part of the way we achieve those types of health is by being in community with others. So, yes, that girls' night out is an important part of balanced, healthy living. Score!

However, just because you're going out to socialize and are getting out of your normal cook-and-clean routine (we all need to get away from that from time to time!) doesn't mean you are leaving your healthy eating habits at home as well. I am NOT saying you have to go out with your friends and watch them dig into fries and cake while you order the plain grilled chicken breast with a side of iceberg. No way! I'd rather stay home!

What I am suggesting is that with a little planning and know-how you can eat delicious food at your favorite restaurant and not break the calorie bank. I suggest limiting yourself to eating out no more than twice per week—and yes, the drive-through and takeout count as eating out, too. This way, you'll have more money to spend on that fresh, real food that you'll be eating throughout the rest of the week, and since you are keeping the number of times that you go out to a minimum, you don't have to obsess over calories and can enjoy yourself more.

You can eat out and enjoy yourself without going crazy and still be able to lose weight. You need to be informed when you're at a restaurant so you can make healthy choices and can splurge intentionally on what you want, not accidentally because you don't know how something is prepared. So commit to asking the questions up front to avoid surprises. It never ceases to amaze me how often healthy-sounding dishes are actually loaded with butter or other fattening ingredients. The only way you can know for sure how a dish is prepared is to ask, and then, if needed, you can request a change or substitution.

When it comes down to it, even when eating out, you can still follow those four components of a flavorful, balanced meal that I told you about right from the get-go:

➤ **Fill half your plate with fruits and/or veggies.**
   ➤ *Try starting your meal with a small salad instead of a traditional appetizer.*
   ➤ *If your dish comes prepared with veggies (like a pasta with veggies in it or a sandwich with veggies as a topping), ask for extra veggies to be added to it. If it doesn't, order a veggie dish as one of your sides.*
   ➤ *If you want dessert, order fresh berries or fruit salad.*
➤ **Fill a quarter of your plate with lean protein.**

5 QUESTIONS YOU SHOULD ASK YOUR WAITER

Your waiter may be the person who can help you make a menu selection that is both tasty and healthy, if you know what to ask. Here are my top 5 questions:

1 **Are there any lighter options on the menu?** Waiters are often used to health-conscious customers, so they're probably familiar with the healthier options. Also, since they know what goes on in the kitchen and how things are prepared, they may be able to advise you on the best choice for your waistline.

2 **What's the most popular dish?** Let's face it—the most popular dish is probably one of the most delicious. Waiters are the perfect people to ask about that, since they're the ones putting in the orders. Plus, they may even dish out their personal favorite option, too! Just don't be afraid to tweak it to make it a little lighter!

3 **What comes on the side?** Menus can be confusing sometimes, and it's important to know what exactly comes with the dish to ensure that it's a healthy choice and to save money! Once you know what comes on the side, you can go ahead and make healthy substitutions. There's no need to order an extra side of brown rice or steamed veggies if you can just substitute something already on the plate.

4 **How big is this meal?** Waiters are usually pretty honest about portion sizes. Sometimes you'll even find that there are cheaper (and healthier) appetizers that would be the perfect size for an entrée! If a dish is big enough to share,

(Continued)

it's better to know that ahead of time so you can plan. Also, if you know it's meant for two, you'll be less likely to eat the whole thing when it arrives at your table.

5 **How is the meal prepared?** It's better to know ahead of time if your dish is fried, grilled, baked, or poached, and if the sides are going to come out covered in a buttery sauce. The waiter can go into more depth than the menu does. It's important to ask your waiter how a dish is prepared even if the menu includes a picture or description of the item. Remember, you may not be able to see added oil in a picture or know what a "flavorful sauce" actually means. So be specific with your questions, and if you do find out that extra fat is added, ask that the chef skip it when he prepares your dish.

> ➤ Grilled fish and poultry are usually great choices; just be aware of added fats and sauces.
> ➤ For beef and pork, the words "loin" and "round" are clues that it is a lean cut (so choose the tenderloin or sirloin instead of the rib eye, for instance).
> ➤ Ask for a half portion, lunch portion, or "petite" version of your meat, poultry, or fish. If that isn't available, remember that a portion should be about the size of your palm for meat or chicken or the size of a checkbook for fish. If it's larger than that, you may want to pack up half of it for later.

➤ **Fill a quarter of your plate with a starch.**
> ➤ Choose either whole grains (brown rice, quinoa, whole-wheat bread, etc.) or starchy veggies (beans, corn, etc.) as your starch whenever possible.
> ➤ Your starch portion should be about the size of a baseball. If it is larger than that, take the rest home.

> ➤ *Ask your server how the starch is prepared (i.e., is butter added to the whole-wheat pasta?) so that you can request changes to the preparation method, if needed.*

➤ **Season your meal with healthy fats, herbs, and spices.**

> ➤ *Ask your server how your meal will be prepared and seasoned. Request that your dish be prepared without added fats for flavor and ask for extra herbs or spices instead. For example, if your server says your grilled steak is finished with a pat of butter, ask that the chef skip the butter and add an extra grind or two of fresh black pepper.*

> ➤ *Try to avoid more than two added fats in your meal. In other words, if you have butter on your baked potato and cheese on your salad, skip the sour cream and bacon on the potato.*

> ➤ *Ask that any added fats (salad dressing, sour cream, cheeses, sauces, etc.) be served on the side so that you can use just a small amount. A little of these items goes a long way when it comes to adding flavor.*

On the days when you eat out for dinner, you may want to have your daily snack an hour or two before going out. That healthy snack will help prevent you from overeating or going gangbusters on the bread basket as soon as you sit down at the restaurant.

In terms of beverages, water is always the best choice. It's free, it has no calories, and therefore it won't add the unwanted, unfilling liquid calories that beverages often include. Speaking of liquid calories—I would not recommend drinking alcohol, especially when you are trying to lose weight. Not only can alcohol impair your ability to make healthy choices, but it also changes the way your body uses calories.

Alcohol contains 7 calories per gram, and when you drink any type of alcohol, your body has to process it right away, meaning it switches to burning those calories first. Any other calories you have consumed, whether from beverages or food, which your body would've been burning off if you weren't drinking, are stored as fat. Alcohol also affects the hormones that regulate hunger and satiety, giving you the perception that you're still hungry, even when you have eaten plenty. That's why it's extra hard to resist the bread basket after you've had a drink.

You will lose weight faster and more efficiently if you abstain from alcohol altogether. Not only will you avoid the consequences mentioned above, but you will also skip the empty calories found in many cocktails. For example, common cocktails like piña coladas, margaritas, and Long Island ice tea can have more than 600 unnourishing, unfilling calories per glass!

But I get it that having a drink from time to time is a part of many people's lifestyle, and this plan allows for individual preferences. So if you are going to have your happy hour drink no matter what I tell you, then be sure to count it as your daily treat. Stick to one glass of wine, a light beer, or a mixed drink made with a calorie-free option like diet soda or club soda so it will fit into your 150-calories-per-day treat budget. The Academy of Nutrition and Dietetics recommends that women have no more than one drink per day for health reasons.

When it comes to eating out, instead of thinking quantity, think quality. Another benefit of going out less often is that when you do go out, you can go to a nicer place!

Below, I have outlined some tasty and better-for-you options at a few of my favorite kinds of restaurants. *Bon appétit!*

Mexican

➤ **Skip the taco salad,** which may sound healthy but usually consists of iceberg lettuce, meat, and loads of cheese and sour cream in a fried tortilla. Opt for another kind of salad if available, or ask for the cheese and sour cream to be served on the side.

➤ **Portion out your tortilla chips.** Instead of eating them straight from the basket, count out 10 chips and put them on your plate.

➤ **Go for corn tortillas** instead of flour tortillas. They have less fat and calories and twice the fiber.

➤ **If you're ordering enchiladas, go for chicken** instead of cheese or ground beef (they usually use the fattier beef rather than lean beef) for a lower-calorie option. Skip the side of rice and beans and order extra peppers and onions instead.

➤ **Pass up the refried beans**, which are loaded with salt and often with fat as well. Order regular black beans instead.

➤ **Load up on the salsa!** It's super low in calories and adds flavor to any dish. Guacamole is another delicious and healthy way to add creaminess to your salad instead of sour cream—just be mindful of your portion size.

➤ **Say no to chimichangas!** They're deep-fried and packed with about 1,200 calories—definitely not worth the splurge!

➤ **Pass on the nachos**, which are essentially more than 1,000 calories of chips loaded with fattening ingredients. Try a tostada instead.

➤ **If ceviche is on the menu, order it** for a satisfying appetizer! It's a low-cal, protein-packed way to start the meal, made with fresh shrimp, veggies, and lime juice.

➤ **Mole sauce is a healthy, delicious sauce** that complements any dish. It's made with peppers, spices, and antioxidant-rich chocolate.

➢ **Flan is a traditional custard** made from milk, eggs, and sugar. It has about the same nutritional content as ice cream, so eat a small portion if you're ordering it for dessert.

Italian

➢ **Order an appetizer featuring fresh seafood**, such as mussels. They tend to be low in calories and fat but packed with flavor.
➢ **Ask for whole-wheat pasta** instead of white pasta.
➢ **Avoid the oily breading** of chicken or eggplant parmigiana. Ask for grilled chicken or eggplant topped with tomato sauce and fresh mozzarella instead.
➢ **When it comes to sauces:**
  ➢ *Choose marinara. It's loaded with an antioxidant called lycopene and is virtually fat-free.*
  ➢ *Pesto sauces are often high in fat due to the large amounts of pine nuts, Parmesan, and olive oil. Though much of the fat is the heart-healthy type, you're better off asking for pesto on the side so you can control your portion size.*
  ➢ *Alfredo sauces (the white, creamy kind) are packed with saturated fat from heavy cream, butter, and Parmesan. Avoid them at all costs!*
➢ **Pass on the Italian sodas.** They usually have just as much sugar as the conventional kind.
➢ **When it comes to dessert, go for a small cannoli** (a typical Italian pastry stuffed with sweetened ricotta) instead of the highly caloric tiramisu. Better yet, share it with a friend! A small scoop of gelato, which is lower in fat since it's made with milk instead of cream, is a good dessert pick as well. Stick to one scoop, because though it's lower in fat than ice cream, it can often be higher in sugar.

Steak House

➤ **Stick to healthier appetizers** like light salads, broth-based soups, and shrimp cocktail. Pass on the fried wings, potato skins, and loaded fries.

➤ **When choosing your steak,** go for leaner cuts like sirloin or tenderloin. Cuts that include "loin" or "round" in the name are usually lean. Strip steaks and skirt steaks are also lean cuts.

➤ **Aim to order a steak** that is around 5 to 6 ounces in size, or if the steaks only come in larger sizes, like 12 ounces, for instance, have the waiter box up half of it before he even brings it out to you. Then you can enjoy the leftovers later.

➤ **Avoid wedge salads.** They're usually nutritionally void iceberg lettuce, bacon, and heavy blue cheese dressing.

➤ **If potatoes are on your mind,** opt for half of a baked potato and add your own toppings instead of ordering a huge pile of mashed potatoes doused in butter and cream. The healthiest side dishes include steamed broccoli, broiled tomatoes, and sautéed spinach (instead of creamed). Asparagus is another good side choice, but make sure to skip the hollandaise!

➤ **When it comes to sauces,** try to avoid béarnaise. The butter and egg yolk sauce will surely sabotage your waistline-friendly meal. Instead try a salsa or a chimichurri sauce.

➤ **Opt for a whole steak** instead of a steak burger, which tends to be made from higher-fat meat.

Greek

➤ **Dolmades** are grape leaves stuffed with rice, spices, and sometimes lamb. One or two (depending on size) are a great way to start off your meal.

➤ **Hummus (made with chickpeas) and baba ghanoush (made**

KEY WORDS TO LOOK FOR OR AVOID ON MENUS

Descriptions of food items on menus are designed to make the food sound tasty, not necessarily to reveal how healthy or unhealthy it might be. However, if you know these key words, you will be able to pick out the menu item that is nutritious and also sounds delicious to you!

These words are tasty green lights when you see them on the menu:

AL FORNO: This is the Italian term describing a dish cooked in the oven. While cooking something in the oven doesn't necessarily ensure that it is healthy, at least it lets you know what method was used to prepare your dish. For example, choosing something that is made *al forno* is usually a better choice than something *fritta*, which means "fried."

GRILLED: Of course, grilling is a healthy cooking method. Just be sure to ask that any additional butter not be added to your dish, as restaurants often top grilled meats with a large pat of butter before serving.

VEGETARIAN: Going meatless when you eat out can help you cut calories and increase your vegetable servings. Just be mindful of ingredients like cheese, which can be overloaded in veggie fare.

RED SAUCE: Whether a marinara sauce at an Italian place or an enchilada sauce at a Mexican joint, red sauces are nearly always healthier than their creamy white counterparts.

When you see menu items described with words in the following list, it's a signal that these items should be saved for special occasions:

CRISPY: Usually this is just a code word for breaded and fried.

CREAMY: This is a signal that lots of butter and/or cream was used to make the dish. Skip it, and select naturally creamy foods like avocados or yogurt instead.

FRITTER: These bad boys are always fried, and the fillings aren't usually the healthiest either.

AU GRATIN: Even if the dish is a vegetable, like spinach or potatoes, the words "au gratin" in front of it on the menu mean it's crusted with cheese, bread crumbs, and butter.

with roasted eggplant) are both delicious and healthy dips. Share them with the table and ask for fresh veggies for dipping instead of gorging on pita.

➤ **Steer clear of pastitsio and moussaka.** Pastitsio, or Greek lasagna, usually consists of loads of pasta with ground beef and a creamy white béchamel sauce. Moussaka is meat, veggies, and the cream sauce. Both score high in fat and calories, thanks to the thick sauce.

➤ **Souvlaki, or kebabs of chicken, beef, pork, or lamb**, are a good entrée choice that often comes with lots of veggies. Pair them with some hummus and a couple small pieces of pita for a complete meal!

➤ **Greek salads** loaded with fresh vegetables like cucumbers, tomatoes, and peppers may sound healthy, but they're usually loaded with feta cheese as well and doused in oily dressing. To make it healthier, order the feta on the side and ask for tzatziki sauce instead. The combo of yogurt, cucumber, and garlic won't weigh you down nearly as much. Just make sure it's made the authentic way with yogurt, not with sour cream!

➤ **Greek restaurants often offer a variety of tasty seafood options.** These are a great high-protein choice, but choose fish that's pan-seared, grilled, or broiled instead of fried. Order veggies on the side instead of the white rice.

- ➤ **Baklava** is a classic Greek dessert made with honey, butter, nuts, and phyllo dough. If you just have to have some, stick to a small piece!

Asian

- ➤ **Ask the waiter to go light on the sugary and salty sauces.** To make veggie-packed stir-fries a good option, request that only a small amount of oil be used in preparation.
- ➤ **Sushi is a great healthy option** that's typically low in fat and usually packed with fresh veggies. Steer clear of the rolls with tempura, cream cheese, and mayonnaise-based sauces. Ask for brown rice instead of white and don't go overboard on the soy sauce.
- ➤ **Stick to a half portion of steamed rice.** It's definitely better than fried, but it'll still add 200 calories to your meal.
- ➤ **Avoid sweet-and-sour chicken, sesame chicken, and General Tso's chicken.** The meat in these dishes is usually deep-fried and then doused in a sugary sauce.
- ➤ **Order kung pao chicken** instead, which comes with abundant vegetables, sans the fried chicken!
- ➤ **Avoid cashew chicken**, which usually consists of fried chicken, oyster sauce, and a handful of cashews.
- ➤ **Ask for extra broccoli, carrots, or snow peas in any dish—** three veggies that Asian restaurants typically have on hand.
- ➤ **Pass on the deep-fried egg rolls.** Each small roll has about 200 calories.
- ➤ **Order a bowl of wonton soup** instead, which is low in calories and will help curb your hunger.

- ➤ **Try steamed pot stickers** for another good appetizer option.
- ➤ **Go for a dish made with grilled tofu or shrimp** to keep your protein lean.
- ➤ **Pass on the high-calorie lo mein dishes**, which include tons of noodles dripping in sauce.
- ➤ **Look for steamed dishes**, such as steamed shrimp with vegetables, which is surprisingly flavorful and dodges all that added oil, too!

Fast/Casual Food

- ➤ **Be smart about salad.** Vegetables are great, but with creamy dressings, calories and fat grams can really add up fast. Vinaigrettes and low-fat dressings are healthier choices. Also beware of toppings such as cheeses and meats, which can easily increase calorie and fat content! Keep it light!
- ➤ **Think grilled, lean meats.** Grilled fish or chicken sandwiches are both good choices. A veggie burger is a healthy meat-free choice. Steer clear of the fried (sometimes called "crispy") chicken, bacon or large-size burgers, as they have a higher calorie and saturated fat content.
- ➤ **Request whole-wheat bread** when ordering sandwiches, burgers, or wraps. Lots of restaurants have these options but don't list them on the menu.
- ➤ **Ask that your burger or sandwich be wrapped in a lettuce leaf** if the bread is massive or there is no whole-wheat bread available.
- ➤ **Skip the extra-large fries and the Big Gulp Coke.** One 32-oz. Big Gulp of regular cola packs about 425 calories (and remember, we are shooting for 450 calories in your whole meal!). Instead of the large fries, how about a baked potato?

But be careful not to ruin this healthy choice by loading it with sour cream, butter, bacon, and other fatty toppings. Instead, top it with salsa, mustard, or a low-fat dressing.

➢ **Nix the cheese on the sandwich** (it probably already has plenty of fat). Instead, top it with some extra pickles, onions, lettuce, and tomato to add flavor and nutrition. It is also a good idea to skip the mayonnaise and high-fat "special sauces" on your sandwich. Ask for ketchup and other condiment packets on the side, and that way you will be able to control the amount used.

➢ **Say no to supersizing.** An average fast-food meal can add up to 1,000 calories or more! So choose a smaller portion size, order a side salad instead of fries, and don't supersize anything!

Now you can dine out at any restaurant you want this weekend without blowing the healthy choices you made this week!

I like to be an informed consumer, so I think it's great that more and more restaurants are providing nutritional information for their menu items. I encourage you to take advantage of this information during your 10 minutes of meal planning each week. If you know at the beginning of the week where you'll be dining out, take 2 minutes to look up the menu and plan your healthy order. Remember to stick close to the 450-calorie guideline for lunch and dinner. When you look up the restaurant's nutritional information, be sure to note whether it pertains to the whole dish or half the dish. Many times restaurants will list a side dish or an entrée as two or more servings, even if it is presented as one dish.

Forgot to look up the menu online? Use a free smartphone app like My Fitness Pal to check the calories right before you order.

Remember though, weight loss and good nutrition are not just about counting calories. They are about making calories count as well. So take stock of your meal as a whole, keeping your balanced meal pattern in mind, and look for dishes that are not only lower in calories but also higher in protein, healthy fats, and fiber.

Some restaurants don't have nutritional information available. In those situations, is it really possible to make a somewhat healthy choice? While meals enjoyed out are almost never as nutritious and calorie-controlled as meals you can make at home, I do think that it is possible to make the best choices wherever you're dining if you make use of the following key strategies.

I developed these strategies because I love supporting local eateries, but oftentimes those are the very places that don't have nutritional information available. So these simple tips have helped me to enjoy my favorite restaurants without packing on the pounds, and they can do the same for you!

➤ **Go halfies from the get-go.** You already know that restaurant portions are generous—way bigger than they should be—and even though you may have every good intention to eat just half of your order, research shows that once food is on the plate, we are probably going to eat it. Instead, when you place your order, ask the waiter to go ahead and pack half of your meal in a to-go container before he brings it out to you. Instant, easy portion control.

➤ **Keep it simple with sides.** Stick to sides that are prepared in a simple way, like grilled or steamed. Some studies have found that specialty side dishes are often higher in calories and fat than some entrées, so keep it simple. Need ideas? I often ask for a fresh sliced tomato in the summertime or a baked sweet potato with cinnamon in the winter.

➤ **Be wary of the use of certain colors and shapes.** Many restaurants use red and yellow in their decor or on the menu, as studies have shown that these colors can help stimulate the appetite. Restaurants will also put specials or high-dollar items in boxes or denote them with a star to catch your eye.

And since our eyes tend to naturally fall to the top right-hand side of a menu, they may put the item they want you to order in this area. So read the menu carefully to make sure you aren't ordering a dish just because it's printed in red or in an eye-catching position.

➢ **Decide if it's really a deal.** A restaurant may offer a special price for a combo or have a prix fixe menu with several courses to entice you to order more. However, decide if you would be just as satisfied without those extras. If so, the offering really isn't a deal for you, and you're better off just sticking to an entrée to save money and calories. Usually what I tell clients is that if you are going to have an appetizer, don't have a dessert too. Either way, you should split those courses and count it as your treat for the day.

With a little planning and asking the right questions, you can enjoy your two meals out per week without seeing your weight loss slow down at all! Who knows? In the process of making healthier restaurant choices, you may discover some delicious dishes you never knew existed! Making healthier choices—even small ones—can truly change the way you look and feel. To feel even better, keep reading to find out how you can gain the lasting energy that you need to power through even your busiest days.

CHAPTER 8

ENERGIZE YOUR DAY THE HEALTHY WAY

If you find yourself dragging every afternoon, that's probably a sign that you are not fueling your body with nutrient- and vitamin-rich foods that promote stable energy levels. What and how we eat are directly related to how energetic we feel throughout the day.

To understand this process, you need to know what "energy" actually is. Calories are the simplest form of energy. While it's true that most people get more than enough calories each day, it's how we distribute them over the course of a day that can be a problem. That's because when you skip a meal or snack, it causes your body to conserve, instead of use, its energy, which means your metabolism slows down.

Your metabolism is like a fire; if you don't put wood on a fire, after a while it will burn out. Likewise, if you go longer than four hours without eating, your metabolism will slow down and your blood sugar will drop, both of which cause your energy levels to plummet. Try to make sure that you are evenly distributing your calories among three meals and a snack and treat, as outlined by your meal pattern. And make sure to eat a meal or snack at least every four hours.

When you are feeling low on energy, you may find yourself craving sugary snacks or soft drinks, but don't give in. While these may give you a quick energy fix, after the spike, your blood sugar will take a nosedive that will leave you with even less energy than before.

I have designed each of your meals and snacks to include a combination of both carbohydrates and protein/healthy fats to give you maximum energy return. This is because carbohydrates, our bodies' first source of energy, provide energy quickly. When healthy fats and proteins are eaten with carbs, they help that energy to be released at a slower and steadier rate. This helps to avoid a blood sugar spike that leads to an energy crash.

The colorful fruits and veggies in your meal pattern are also important in keeping energy levels up, since some nutrients commonly found in produce can help your body use energy more efficiently. For example, potassium, which is found in veggies like broccoli and potatoes, and in fruits like oranges and bananas, helps to convert the calories from food you eat into energy that your body can use. Magnesium, found in foods such as spinach, beans, and peas, promotes consistent energy levels since it helps to stabilize blood sugar levels in the body.

The B vitamins, found in foods like eggs, leafy greens, whole grains, and legumes, also play a critical role in energy metabolism. B-complex vitamins fuel the brain by helping to metabolize car-bohydrates; a deficiency in these can lead to serious fatigue. Following your meal plan with a balance of fruits, vegetables, whole grains, and lean meats is a surefire way to have adequate intake of the B-complex vitamins.

If you're feeling fatigued, especially during exercise, make sure your zinc levels are adequate. Zinc is essential for all of the enzymes involved in energy metabolism, so low zinc levels can leave you feeling sluggish. You can find it in foods such as milk, lean beef, chicken, beans, and nuts. It's critical for healthy hair, skin, bones, and overall physical well-being.

Research shows a strong correlation between depression and low levels of omega-3 fatty acids. Because chronic fatigue syndrome often goes hand in hand with depression, it's important to consume plenty of omega-3 fats to boost energy and fight fatigue. Get your dose by consuming oily fish like sardines, mackerel, salmon, and tuna as well as plant sources like flaxseed.

Vitamin C is a potent immune-boosting antioxidant, but it also plays a key role in enhancing energy when it comes to physical performance. Fruits like kiwis, oranges, and strawberries or veggies like bell peppers are chock-full of this stuff, so get chomping to minimize muscle weakness and fatigue. Quick tip: Vitamin C also helps aid the absorption of iron!

Iron-deficiency anemia is one of the leading nutritional problems among women. Symptoms include fatigue and weakness, especially during exercise. Iron helps to carry the oxygen in your blood to your brain and your muscles. Without enough oxygen, you'll feel energy-depleted and could even be at risk of passing out. Clearly, getting enough iron in your diet is important! In fact, a study from Cornell University found that active women with low levels of iron suffer symptoms similar to those experienced by women who are actually deficient in iron, such as being slower and weaker.

I experienced this for myself as a collegiate cross-country runner. I falsely believed that by cutting certain foods out of my diet, I would become a leaner and faster runner. Unfortunately, many of the foods that I avoided, like red meat, were good sources of iron. Eventually I started to have trouble completing my runs and was always sapped of energy no matter how much sleep I got. When I went to the doctor,

IRON-RICH FOODS

- Fish and shellfish—tuna, salmon, oysters, clams, shrimp
- Lean meats—beef, pork, lamb
- Poultry—chicken and turkey (dark meat has more than light meat)
- Beans and legumes—kidney, black, soy, pinto, navy, garbanzo, lentils
- Tofu and soy-based meat alternatives like veggie burgers, tempeh
- Greens—spinach, kale; mustard, collard, and turnip greens
- Vegetables—broccoli, asparagus, parsley, Brussels sprouts, potatoes, peas
- Dried fruits—raisins, dates, prunes, apricots
- Iron-fortified whole grains—cereals, breads, tortillas, rice, pasta
- Other—blackstrap molasses, egg yolks, nuts

*Note: Some types of iron-rich foods are more easily absorbed than others. Heme iron, found only in animal foods (meats, poultry, fish), is about twice as well absorbed as nonheme iron (from plant sources). However, you can increase the body's absorption of iron from plant foods by consuming them with foods high in vitamin C. For example, you could put orange slices on your spinach salad to increase absorption of the iron in the spinach.

he diagnosed me with iron-deficiency anemia and sent me to see a registered dietitian, who helped me learn to eat a more balanced diet that included iron-rich foods (like the ones listed on the left). I was so inspired by the connection between what we eat and how we feel that I changed my major and became a dietitian.

Now, as a registered dietitian, I understand that food does not just help us gain or lose weight but also fuels our bodies. When we get plenty of nutrients, like the ones mentioned above, it helps us to keep our energy levels strong.

Just as with weight loss, *when* you eat can be just as important as *what* you eat for maintaining energy levels. If you feel like snoozing after lunch every day, that may mean your meal isn't balanced. A large, high-fat meal will take longer to digest, meaning that blood will stay concentrated in your intestinal tract rather than in your brain, where it helps to keep you alert. That's why it's important to follow your meal pattern. The balance of carbohydrates, protein, and healthy fats provides both quick and long-lasting energy for your afternoon.

Another reason for afternoon energy drain is going too long without eating. Remember that if your lunch and dinner are spaced more than four hours apart, you should have your daily snack in the midafternoon. For lasting energy, make your daily snack one of the energy-boosting snacks from the breakout box on the right.

Drinking plenty of water throughout the day is also important for maintaining high energy levels, as even slight dehydration can cause a decrease in energy. Staying hydrated is without a doubt one of the most important components of overall health and during physical activity, and studies have found that drinking water, especially as opposed to sugary beverages, may help to promote weight loss.

Keep in mind that when it's super hot or cold outside, your body uses more water to maintain its normal temperature, so you may have to up your fluid intake. Also, make sure to properly hydrate before, during, and after working out. Strenuous exercise leads to fluid losses through sweating and breathing, and it's vital that those fluids be replaced. Dehydration is dangerous and can lead to nasty side effects like dizziness, lethargy, and cramping. To avoid dehydration, drink 15–20 ounces of water a couple of hours before exercise. Every 15–20 minutes during exercise, it's recommended to drink about 8–10 ounces. To ensure that you're getting enough water, carry a reusable water bottle with you throughout the day. It's a constant reminder to drink up!

A moderate amount of caffeine is okay to provide a quick fix for your afternoon pick-me-up. In fact, some studies have linked moderate caffeine consumption from coffee and green tea to weight loss and healthy weight maintenance. This may be because caffeine

ENERGY-BOOSTING SNACKS

1 6 Triscuits + 1 tbsp. almond butter

2 ¼ cup hummus + 1 sliced bell pepper

3 1½ cups air-popped popcorn + 1 oz. dark chocolate

4 1 slice whole-grain toast + ½ sliced banana + 2 tsp. peanut butter + dash of cinnamon

5 1 medium pear + string cheese

6 6 oz. nonfat Greek yogurt + ½ cup berries + 2 tbsp. slivered almonds

7 ¼ cup raw almonds sprinkled with cocoa powder and stevia + ½ cup grapes

8 ¾ cup low-fat cottage cheese with 8 strawberries

9 3 tbsp. guacamole + 12 baked tortilla chips

10 1 brown rice cake + 1 tbsp. whipped cream cheese + 2 oz. smoked salmon

HOW MUCH WATER IS ENOUGH?

Did you know you lose about 10 cups of water per day through normal body functions alone, like sweating and breathing? So how much water is enough? Contrary to the popular belief of aiming for eight glasses a day, it is now recommended that healthy adults actually use thirst to determine their needs. According to the 2004 Institute of Medicine guidelines, women should be drinking about 91 ounces of fluids per day, or about 11 cups. This recommendation includes total water intake, from both food and beverages. Assuming that 80% of our fluids come from water and 20% come from food, it's a safe bet to recommend that women drink about 9 cups of water daily. Meeting 20% of your fluid needs from food may seem like a lot to shoot for, but foods like grapefruit, watermelon, and lettuce are more than 90% water!

seems to suppress leptin, a hormone that affects the appetite. Research has also shown that having a cup of java before you work out may help you to be able to exercise both harder and longer, as caffeine may block signals of muscle fatigue. The bottom line is that for the majority of healthy adults, it's completely safe to have two to three cups of java daily, or at most 300 milligrams of caffeine a day (see the chart about caffeine content to see how much caffeine you're consuming each day). And contrary to what you've probably heard, you can't become addicted to your morning cup of joe. That said, you may still notice some short-term symptoms if you habitually drink caffeine and suddenly stop.

But don't get too much of a good thing! Excessive caffeine consumption may lead to some adverse health effects, such as

CAFFEINE CONTENT OF COMMON FOODS

Item	Item Size	Caffeine (mg)
Coffee	5 oz.	60–150
Decaf coffee	5 oz.	2–5
Tea	5 oz.	40–80
Hot chocolate	5 oz.	1–8
Espresso	1 oz.	75
Starbucks Tall Brewed Coffee	12 oz.	260
Starbucks Tall Caramel Macchiato	12 oz.	75
Starbucks Tall Caffé Latte	12 oz.	75
Starbucks Tall Caffé Mocha	12 oz.	95
Starbucks Tall Frappuccino	12 oz.	70
Starbucks Tall Caffé Americano	12 oz.	150
Monster X-presso	6.8 oz.	221
Red Bull Energy Drink	8.4 oz.	83
Amp Energy	8 oz.	71
Diet Coca-Cola	12 oz.	45
Chocolate brownie	1.25 oz.	8
Milk chocolate	1 oz.	1–15

increased blood pressure and heart problems, especially in those with hypertension. Plus, drinking too much caffeine can make you feel anxious and cause insomnia, which of course will deplete your energy faster than you can say, "Make mine a double espresso."

Not only does lack of sleep affect your energy levels, but it can also lead to weight gain. Harvard scientists found that people who sleep for less than five hours a night are much more likely to gain weight over the course of a year than people who sleep a full seven hours. Perhaps this is because when your body is low on energy from not getting enough sleep, you may be more likely to turn to your next most readily available source of energy: food in the form of simple sugar.

If you are not in the habit of getting at least seven hours of sleep, start working in that direction. Try to go to bed 15 minutes earlier each night until you reach the seven-hour mark. Once you hit that goal, find a bedtime that works well for you (aiming for between seven and nine hours of sleep) and stick to that time. Going to bed at the same time every night will result in higher-quality sleep, which means more energy, and will aid you in making better food choices.

If you have trouble falling asleep at night you may want to try the following tips:

➤ Turn off the TV, computer, and all other electronics at least 30 minutes before bed. The bright light from these devices can cause your brain to stay awake. Instead, do something relaxing: take a warm bath, read your favorite book or magazine, say a prayer, or meditate to help you wind down for the evening.

➤ If you have trouble falling asleep because your brain is "running," thinking about all the things you have to do or what tomorrow is going to be like, keep a pad of paper and a pen by your bed and write these things down. This action will help switch your brain to "off."

➤ Try eating your daily snack at bedtime and enjoy one of the sleep-inducing munchies from the breakout box in Chapter 3.

➤ Avoid exercising within four hours of bedtime. While exercise can certainly boost your energy levels, you don't want to be on an energy high when you are trying to fall asleep at night.

Even though you may want to avoid exercise before bed, it is still important to work exercise into your day. Not only does it naturally boost energy levels; it will also improve your overall health, boost your mood, and help you lose weight faster. I recommend a minimum of 30 minutes of exercise every day for weight loss and weight maintenance; however, if you want to lose weight even faster and more effectively, shoot for an hour of physical activity per day.

You may be thinking, "Umm, sorry, but I bought this book because I am so busy that I barely have time to eat healthy, much less exercise." Don't freak out just yet! You don't have to fit all 30–60 minutes into one session. In fact, studies show that three 10-minute exercise sessions are just as effective as one 30-minute session. So you could power walk for 10 minutes during your morning coffee break (come on, I know you spend at least that much time on Facebook; just trade that in for a spin around the office), 10 minutes during your lunch break, and 10 minutes when you get off work.

 ## REAL-LIFE SUCCESS STORY

learned the trick of filling half my plate with vegetables and the rest with other foods. I also learned that I need someone to hold me accountable regularly for me to reach my health and fitness goals. Sarah-Jane encouraged me to try a new fitness class I had been interested in but had never tried before, Pure Barre. I decided to do it and now, over a year later, I am addicted! Watching my body change really motivated me for the first time in years. The best results for me personally were dropping my body fat by 10% and gaining the confidence to feel like I could succeed. Simple tools and small changes can make a big difference. It can help you curb weight gain and start losing.

—*Libby B.*

TIP FROM LIBBY: If you start feeling overwhelmed with changing your whole lifestyle, break it down into smaller pieces. Rather than always looking at the big picture, simply focus on each individual snack or meal opportunity as it arises and try to make the best choice possible in that moment.

You can also work exercise into your day if you can't carve out specific space for it. Try these ways to squeeze physical activity into your schedule. Keep track of your minutes so you can be sure to hit the 30–60 mark.

- Park farther away from the office to add some walking to your daily commute.
- Take the stairs instead of the elevator every time you have the choice.
- Walk the halls during phone calls or schedule walking meetings with colleagues.
- Instead of driving through the drugstore, dry cleaners, etc., park your car and walk in.
- Wear a pedometer and aim to take 10,000 steps per day.
- Try some of the strength-building exercises in the "Squeezing Exercise In" breakout box that allow you to exercise while doing your normal daily tasks.

When it comes to exercise, if you are more the hit-it-hard-and-get-it-done-fast type, you can always go to the gym for a major sweat session of spin class or treadmill intervals, but on days when you don't have time for that, try this lunchtime calorie crusher. Simply

SQUEEZING EXERCISE IN

These strength and toning exercises won't take any additional time from your day, but they are still effective. Please note that for maximum results, you should combine them with some form of cardio activity as well, such as walking, jogging, or biking.

- Every time you brush your teeth do calf raises. Steady yourself by placing the hand you are not using to brush your teeth on the bathroom counter. Then come up on your tiptoes and back down to flat-footed. Repeat until you are done brushing your teeth, 1–2 minutes.
- When you are waiting for a pot to boil or a dish to finish cooking, try countertop push-ups. Find a clean countertop in your kitchen away from the food that is being prepared and stand facing it with your waist touching the edge of the counter and your hands about shoulder width apart gripping the counter on each side of your body. Take a giant step back with your hands still gripping the counter until your arms are straight. Then line your feet up at about hip width. Lower yourself until your chest almost touches the counter and then push back up until your arms are straight again. Aim for two sets of 12.
- When you are talking on the phone, do squats. Stand with your feet hip width apart and your hand that is not holding the phone extended or holding on to a chair for balance. Then lower yourself as if you were going to sit in a chair, until your upper legs are bent at almost 90 degrees, parallel to the floor, taking care that your knees do not extend over your toes (you should be able to see your toes at all times during this motion—this protects your knees from injury). Repeat this action 20 times for at least two sets.

(Continued)

- While you're working on the computer, try leg raises. Tighten your abdominal muscles while you lift your legs straight up with toes pointed until your toes touch the underside of your desk. Slowly bend your knees and bring your pointed toes back toward the floor, stopping just before they touch it. Go for three sets of eight.
- Before you leave work at the end of the day, rock out a few sets of tricep dips at your desk for great-looking arms. Face away from the desk with your backside on the edge, palms on the top of the desk. Keep your feet together and bend your elbows, putting your weight into your arms, then dip down a few inches off the desk until your elbows form a 90-degree angle. Go for three sets of 15.
- When you're watching TV, take advantage of the commercials by squeezing in some planks for a tight core. Try holding each plank for 45 seconds and increasing your time by 10 seconds each commercial. Get in push-up form and drop to your elbows. Keep your core tight the whole time and make sure not to let hips and butt rise.
- While you're cooking dinner, grab a couple cans of beans or soup for shoulder raises. Start with your arms relaxed at your sides, holding a can in each hand. Raise both of your arms out to the side until they're parallel to the floor. Slowly lower them back down to your sides. Aim for three sets of 10.
- When you get up in the morning, lunge to the bathroom instead of walking to strengthen your legs and butt. Stand straight with your feet shoulder width apart. Step one foot about three feet in front of your body, bending your knee to a right angle. Make sure your knees don't go past your toes! Push off the ground with your right foot until you're back to starting position. Repeat with the other leg. Go for three sets of 10 lunges.

find a flight of stairs during your lunch break and spend the first half of your break walking those stairs. You will burn roughly 300 calories in 30 minutes (based on a body weight of 160 pounds). Not a bad way to sneak in a calorie-busting workout!

If you make these dietary changes, get plenty of sleep, and exercise regularly but still experience low energy levels, you may want to visit your doctor to rule out any medical conditions that could be causing your symptoms.

Not only can food help us lose weight and feel more energetic, but how we eat it can make a difference as well. In Chapter 9, I'll show you that *how* you eat is just as important as *what* you eat.

CHAPTER 9

HOW YOU EAT IS JUST AS IMPORTANT AS WHAT YOU EAT

We've spent a lot of time talking about what to eat to lose weight and have more energy, but *how* you eat can ultimately make or break your success. That's because mindful eaters, people who consume their food at a table without distractions, tend to eat less and still feel more satisfied. This can be especially hard to do when you're busy, so in this chapter I will reveal the benefits of being a mindful eater and give you strategies for eating more mindfully even on the busiest of days.

In general, mindful eaters exhibit four major characteristics:

1. They are able to identify true physical hunger, and they eat only when hungry and stop at the first point of fullness.

2. They eat sitting down at a table.
3. They eat from a plate or a bowl instead of straight out of a bag or box.
4. They eat without distractions (i.e., TV, reading, computer, cell phone).

Whenever you are able, I encourage you to abide by these four principles. It will help you to lose weight and eat less without even trying. In fact, many times at initial meetings with clients, I instruct them not to change anything about what they are eating but rather to change how they are eating for a week. They always come back shocked at how just being more mindful as they eat helps them eat less and feel more satisfied after the meal.

Learn to Identify True Hunger

Being able to identify actual physical hunger and to distinguish it from emotional hunger is truly the first step to becoming a mindful eater. Many of the excess calories we consume are eaten when we are not really physically hungry. We may think we are hungry when we are actually stressed, sad, bored, or tired. We often turn to food to soothe these emotions, but the only thing food can satisfy is true physical hunger. So we eat more and more, trying to feel better, but we end up feeling worse and gaining weight.

To determine whether hunger is physical or emotional, I often encourage clients to do the "apple test." When the munchies strike, simply ask yourself if an apple (or some other food that you feel neutral about) would satisfy the hunger. If the answer is yes, then most likely the hunger is physical hunger. You are truly hungry, so any nourishing food sounds good. If the answer is no, then an emotion is most likely driving the "hunger" you are feeling, creating a specific food craving. That's a good time to evaluate what you are

HOW TO STAY OCCUPIED WHEN YOU THINK YOU'RE HUNGRY

- **Work out!** Pump up your heart rate and listen to music to occupy your mind. Even if it's just a 10-minute walk, you'll likely forget about eating and squeeze in a mini workout, too!
- **Read a book.** Getting caught up in a story will help you forget that you wanted a snack in the first place.
- **Pick up the phone.** If you're an emotional eater, instead of turning to your fork, try calling your best friend instead. Talking about why you're feeling the way you do will satisfy you more than food will.
- **Brush your teeth.** The minty freshness may be all you need to say "no" to mindless munching. Plus, most foods don't taste all that great post-brushing anyway!
- **Have tea time.** Drink a fruity cup of herbal tea for a boost of flavor and comforting warmth sans the calories.
- **Paint your nails.** This is the perfect activity, since you can't very well eat and do a manicure at the same time. Plus, your nails will be too pretty to mess up with food afterward! And who doesn't love a good mani?
- **Organize your junk drawers.** We all have 'em. Spend some time fixing them up for a double-whammy feeling of accomplishment and avoiding mindless snacking.
- **Drink a big glass of water.** Often, thirst disguises itself as hunger. Plus, studies show that drinking water before you eat can help you eat less.
- **Chew gum or suck on a hard candy.** Because we want to eat when we're bored, chewing on something can take your mind off thinking it's hungry and keep your mouth occupied.

truly feeling (stressed, bored, sad, etc.) and find a more effective way to soothe that emotion (check out the breakout box for some ideas). It only takes a second to do the "apple test," and it can help change the way you eat so that you can lose weight and keep it off for good. No matter how busy you are, and even if you are eating on the go, this is one easy mindful-eating strategy that you can do every time before you eat.

Create a Peaceful Dining Experience

Studies show that people eat more when they are standing up than when they are sitting down. And people in a hurry are more likely to eat out of a bag or a box while standing, which means they probably have no way of knowing how much food they actually end up consuming. When you are eating meals and snacks at home, be sure you have a table that is clear of clutter where you can sit down to enjoy your food. Be kind to yourself. You deserve to have a peaceful, enjoyable environment in which to eat. You may even want to enhance the ambience and put out a nice place mat or light a candle.

Sitting down in this kind of setting enables you to focus more on the food you are eating. You will be more aware of the satisfying flavors and textures in your meal, which will help you feel more satisfied. You will also have a better idea of how much you are eating, which will prevent overeating. Just the act of sitting down to eat can help slow down your eating as well, which is a good thing, since it really does take 20 minutes for your brain to know that your stomach is satisfied.

Let's be realistic. I know there will be many meals that you will eat in your office, rushing around in your kitchen, or on the go, but you can still make an effort to do so mindfully. If you are eating a meal at the office, take at least 10–20 minutes to sit and enjoy your food. Clear a space on your desk, or better yet, get out of your work setting and head to the break room or outside to a picnic table. That way, your brain doesn't associate work and stress with eating and later allow those conditions to lead to mindless eating.

Eat from a Plate

Eating from a plate or bowl rather than from a bag or box goes hand in hand with sitting down at a table to eat. Not only does this elevate eating from an animalistic instinct to an enjoyable experience, but it also requires you to portion out the food to put it on the plate, keeping you aware of how much you consume. It also allows you to easily see whether you are following the recommended meal pattern of filling half your plate with fruits and veggies, a fourth of your plate with lean protein, and a fourth of your plate with carbs and seasoning with spices, herbs, and healthy fats.

We eat with our eyes first, so nicely plating your food can really make it more satisfying. If you don't believe me, try eating the Peanut Butter and Berry Yogurt from an elegant martini glass or enjoying the Pan-Glazed Chicken with Kale from a nice china plate. Your meals will be taken to a new level!

When you are ready to eat a meal or snack, serve your plate and then put away any leftovers immediately, before you sit down to eat. This way you will be less likely to grab seconds or thirds just because the food is sitting in front of you. If you are following the meal pattern, you will likely find that you are plenty satisfied without seconds anyway.

I recommend using a salad plate for most of your meals rather than a dinner plate. You'll have instant portion control! Switching to a smaller plate helps you feel more satisfied with less food because you'll be able to enjoy a full plate of food rather than feeling gypped when you see small portions of food on a large plate. And to tell you the truth, modern salad plates are a more appropriate size anyway.

MAKING IT EASIER TO MEASURE PORTIONS

- Get an extra set or two of measuring cups at the dollar store and keep a quarter-cup measure in the package of foods that you commonly consume, such as cereal, nuts, and dried fruit.
- Use a measuring cup to serve food directly from the cooking pot onto your plate rather than using a serving spoon.
- Use clear glass or plastic dishes and cups that have stripes or other designs on them so that you can take note of where in the dish or cup a half-cup or one-cup serving comes to. Or purchase dishes discretely designed for this type of portion control, such as Elegant Portions (http://elegantportions.com/).
- When you buy a large package of food, such as a bag of nuts or a box of crackers, immediately transfer single servings into individual plastic baggies so that they are measured and ready when you are.
- Use a plate that contrasts in color from the food you are eating. So if you are eating mashed potatoes, eat them from a blue plate rather than a white plate. A study from the *Journal of Consumer Research* found that people served themselves a larger portion of food when its color was close to the color of the plate.

The size of dinner plates has increased by about 23% in just the past 20 years. Just take a look at the plates your mother or grandmother may have received as a wedding gift. You may be surprised at just how much smaller than today's plates they really are. Is it any coincidence that America's rates of obesity have increased right along with the size of the plates? Cornell researchers found that just by switching from a 12-inch plate to a 10-inch plate, you could consume up to 22% fewer calories!

When eating from a plate or bowl just simply is not an option, it is crucial that you measure out the correct serving size of each food for your meal or snack. For instance, if you always end up eating breakfast in the car on the way to work, measure out your cereal, nuts, and berries the night before and put them in plastic baggies. The next morning, grab the baggies and an individual serving-sized container of yogurt. Having items already measured is especially important when you are eating on the go because you don't have the visual cues and built-in portion control that a plated meal or snack provides.

Adhering to a healthy diet isn't just about *what* and *how* we eat, but also *how much* we eat. Keeping portion sizes in check is no easy feat. Focus on nutrient-dense foods like lean meat, low-fat dairy, whole grains, and fruits and vegetables instead of processed foods. The more high-quality food you eat, the fuller you'll be and the less packaged food you'll need to satisfy cravings! Also, remember that it takes about 20 minutes for your brain to realize you're full. Try filling your plate up once and then wait a good while before going for seconds.

Though recommended portion sizes are listed on all food labels, it's pretty tough to eyeball a cup of cereal or half a cup of rice without whipping out a measuring cup. Luckily, there are some great shortcuts out there that compare a serving of common foods we eat to everyday objects. Here are a few quick tricks to tackling perfect portion control:

➤ A 3-oz. serving of meat is the size of a deck of cards.
➤ A 5-oz. serving of fish is the size of a checkbook.
➤ A 1-cup serving of pasta is the size of a tennis ball.
➤ 2 tablespoons of butter is the size of a Ping-Pong ball.

- ½ cup of cooked veggies, potatoes, quinoa, or rice is the size of a baseball.
- ¼ cup of dried fruit is the size of a large egg or a golf ball.
- A medium baked potato is the size of a computer mouse.
- A 1-oz. serving of cheese is the size of 6 dice.
- 1 pancake or bread serving is the size of a CD.

Eat Without Distractions

Eating without distractions may be the most important part of mindful eating. Research has proven time and time again that people eat more when they are not solely focused on the food. You may not think that you are very distracted by the TV or by browsing Pinterest on your cell phone as you eat, but you would be surprised. A study from the *American Journal of Clinical Nutrition* reported that people who ate in front of the TV consumed more food and were more likely to describe their meal as unsatisfying as well.

TV isn't the only culprit that distracts us during mealtime. Any activity other than eating or conversing with fellow diners should be avoided to truly have a mindful experience. Work, reading, computers, tablets, phones—all will take our focus away from the food and result in our eating more and enjoying it less. In short, distractions make us remember less about our meal, and the less we remember, the more likely we are to eat more later. And when we are squeezing meals into a busy day, it can be even harder to remember what we ate for lunch. That's why eating at the table is such a good idea; it automatically moves us away from many of these distractors and makes our meals more memorable.

It may feel a little strange to eat in silence if you are used to eating with distractions, but give it a try for a couple of weeks and you will see the difference it makes, I promise. In fact, I work from home and so I eat breakfast and lunch alone nearly every day. I have found that eating mindfully has made such a difference in how I eat that even though I am by myself, I take the time to move away from my computer and eat from a plate at the table whenever possible.

Of course, there are some times when eating without distractions simply isn't an option. Maybe you are running late and have to eat a meal in the car or you have a tight deadline that requires you to work through lunch. The good news is that if you make eating without distractions a habit, you will still be a more mindful eater, even when you can't avoid the distractions. You will likely still eat slower and still be more aware of what and how much you are eating. So for those times that you can't create a fully mindful eating experience, just remember to minimize distractions as much as possible (turn off the music in the car, turn your phone to silent in the office), do the "apple test," and make sure your food is measured out to the correct portion size.

If you want to enjoy your food more and lose weight with little effort, mindful eating is key. Most of these changes in how you eat won't take much time, but they will have a huge impact on your success. As you become a more mindful eater, you will move from viewing eating as a stressful, guilt-ridden experience to regarding it as a peaceful and pleasurable one. And you will be losing weight in the process! It doesn't get much better than that!

Now that you know what, how, and how much you should be eating, in Chapter 10 we'll talk about how to do it for life so that you'll keep the weight off for good!

CHAPTER *10*

BUSIER AND BETTER THAN EVER FOREVER

By now you have seen how the power of planning can work for you. Just 30 minutes per week has enabled you to shed those unwanted pounds, have more energy than you thought was possible, and enjoy meals that truly are both healthy and delicious— all while living your fabulous, busy life!

This is your new lifestyle. Since the plan focuses on moderation, *not* deprivation, you probably won't feel the same temptation to quit that you may have felt with diets in the past. But that, of course, is because this is not a diet, but rather a game plan for success. And now that you have tasted success, you know how sweet it truly is.

That's why I know you will stick with this new lifestyle! My clients can tell you that it is truly realistic, and the secret really is all about the power of planning. They have continued to plan every week and have kept the weight off for years as well. I know you can do it too! You now have the secret. You have a plan, and you even have a Plan B!

That's not to say there won't be challenges along the way. Life happens and brings unplanned challenges with it. Sometimes even the good things in life, like holidays and vacations, can throw your healthy habits into a tailspin. So what happens then?

You simply get up and get back on the horse. In this chapter, I will give you tools to help you get back in the saddle again, should you fall off. It happens to all of us at some point. The first step is to avoid beating yourself up about getting slightly off track. If you do beat yourself up, you are more likely to stay off track than if you take a more positive approach and look at it as a learning experience. It's an opportunity to evaluate the situation, determine what triggered the hiccup in your healthy habits, and plan what to do to prevent it from happening in the future. For example, if you end up raiding the vending machine because you forgot to restock your emergency snack stash during your weekly planning session, you can make a list of what to add to the stash next week and set a reminder on your phone to restock your stash.

If you really take 30 minutes once a week for the power-planning session, mistakes like this won't happen very often. You will have created an environment that makes healthy choices easy. So if you temporarily fall off the horse, get yourself back on it by reinstating your power-planning session that very day.

In addition to planning, one of the things that has helped my clients stay on track, and especially get back on track if they took a detour, is to keep track of what they are eating via a food journal. Research has shown that people who keep a food journal lose twice as much weight as those that don't, even if they are following the same eating plan.

HOW TO KEEP AN EFFECTIVE FOOD JOURNAL

Consider including these items to make food journaling work for you.

- **Time:** Record the time that you eat each meal and snack. This way, you'll be able to evaluate if you are going too long between meals, which can lead to overeating.
- **Hunger Level:** Rate your hunger level before each meal and snack on a scale of 1–10 where 1 is ravenous, 5 is neutral, and 10 is stuffed. Aim to be at a 3–4 when you eat and at a 5–6 when you finish eating. If you find yourself eating when you are not truly hungry, you may need to evaluate why you are eating (stress, boredom, etc.) and find a better solution for dealing with those emotions. On the other hand, if you find yourself regularly eating when you are ravenous, you may want to plan for a snack between meals or space meals no more than 4 hours apart to prevent overeating.
- **Portion Sizes:** Writing down what you eat and drink at each meal and snack is a good start, but recording how much of each food and beverage you consume is important too. Doing this will keep you aware of portion sizes, which is essential for weight loss.
- **Observations:** Include any observations you have after eating the meal or snack. Did the combination of certain textures or flavors make the meal super-satisfying? Did you eat the meal mindfully? Did the meal fill you up or leave you wanting more? Recording this information will be very helpful for planning future meals and snacks.

WHY YOU SHOULD KEEP A FOOD JOURNAL

- Scientists at several clinical research centers in the United States found that dieters who kept a food diary lost twice as much weight as those who didn't. In a six-month study, participants who kept a food journal six or seven days a week lost an average of 18 pounds (8 kilograms), compared with an average of 9 pounds (4 kilograms) lost by those who did not keep a journal.

- The study tracked nearly 1,700 overweight or obese adults across the country who were at least 25 years old. Men and women were included.

- All participants were encouraged to use weight-loss maintenance strategies such as calorie restriction, weekly group sessions, and moderately intensive exercise, as well as to keep a food journal.

You may think you don't have time to keep a food journal, but there are several apps that take the tediousness out of the old-fashioned paper-and-pencil journaling system. The free app My Fitness Pal, for example, has one of the most comprehensive food databases of any program I've seen. This means you can use the app to simply do a keyword search for whatever it is you are eating, whether it is a meal at a restaurant or a recipe you whipped up at home. You'll likely find it; then you can select it and the app will keep a running tally of your calorie count for the day. This will help you stay focused on your goals.

And if even that sounds like it will take too much time, simply use your smartphone to snap a pic of your plate every time you eat. Look through the photos at the end of the day to see if you stuck to our four-part meal pattern (filling half your plate with fruits and veggies, filling a quarter of your plate with a lean protein, filling a quarter of your plate with complex carbs, and using healthy fats, herbs, and spices to season your meal). Just by taking a minute each day to evaluate what you ate, you'll be able to know where you're doing well and what areas need improvement.

One way to improve your habits is to focus on one meal at a time rather than throwing a whole day away because you made one poor choice. A mistake here and there won't derail you from reaching your goals, but throwing whole days or weeks to the wind can. Instead of taking an all-or-nothing approach, look at each meal or snack as an opportunity to make a smart choice. The key to avoiding

THE BEST FOOD-TRACKING APPS

- **My Fitness Pal:** This free app provides a comprehensive database of more than 2,000,000 homemade foods and restaurant items, along with 350 exercises, so you can track your diet and workouts! Compatible with iPhone, Android, Windows, and BlackBerry.

- **Lose It!** This free app helps you set goals for everything from weight loss and exercise to sleep. You can track your progress using the simple interface, and you don't need an Internet connection to use it. Compatible with iPhone, iPod touch, iPad, and Android.

- **MyNetDiary Pro:** For $3.99 this app provides you with a commercial bar code scanner, a recipe editor, weekly analysis (providing tips and advice on overcoming weight plateaus), and more. Compatible with iPhone, iPod touch, iPad, Android, and BlackBerry.

- **Shroomies Nutrition Menu:** *Fitness* magazine deemed this $1.99 app "the mother of all iPhone calorie counters" since the app has the largest nutritional database on the app store (93,000 items, with over 41,000 restaurant items). Compatible with iPhone, iPod touch, and iPad.

- **My Nutrition:** This free app allows users to track their meals with more than 8,000 indexed foods directly from the USDA. The My Family feature calculates recommendations for your whole family to help with meal planning. Compatible with iPhone, iPad, and iPod touch.

- **MealLogger:** This free app allows you to photograph your meals and log your exercise and sends the data to a Web site, where your dietitian can give you feedback online or by text message. Compatible with Android, BlackBerry, iPhone, iPod touch, and iPad. Requires iOS 4.3 or later.

a complete nosedive is to get back on track as soon as possible. As soon as you realize you've made a poor choice or two, jump back to your healthy meal pattern for the very next meal. Don't become a victim of "Monday Syndrome," as I call it, where you fall off the horse, and then say, "Oh well, I'll start over on Monday." There are two problems with this approach. Number one, your unhealthy choices will be prolonged, making it harder to get back on track. And, number two, you miss out on the extra time that weekends often offer, which could be used for a power-planning session to ensure your success for the following week. If you wait until Monday, you'll be thrown into the busy workweek unprepared, which will lead to a whole endless cycle of "off" weeks.

If during one of those "off" weeks, you made some poor choices at the grocery store and your pantry or fridge is now taunting you with chips and ice cream, take some time to reorganize to get back on the right foot. Of course, since you can enjoy one treat daily on the *Schedule Me Skinny* plan, having some of these treat-type foods around is okay. However, when you've been off track, I recommend having no more than two treat foods on hand at any given time. If you find yourself with more than that, toss a couple of items or give them away. Studies show that the more varied foods we have to choose from, the more we'll eat.

You'll also eat more if the treats are easy to spot. This is where organization comes into play. The foods that live at eye level in your pantry or fridge will be the ones that you'll most likely grab first, so keep those chopped veggies and fruits or canned beans at eye level and place treats in the bottom of a dark pantry or in the back of the fridge or freezer. In addition, if you do keep anything out in a bowl on your desk or countertop, make sure it is fresh fruit or veggies rather than candy. The old adage "out of sight, out of mind" really is true.

Eating mindfully is important too. When you have been off track,

ORGANIZED FOR HEALTH

Use these tips to get your kitchen and diet back in order.

- **Strategic Containers:** Store healthy foods at eye level in your fridge or pantry in clear containers so that your eyes will automatically be drawn to the best choices for meal and snack items. Keep treats in opaque containers at the back of the fridge or pantry to keep them out of sight and out of mind.
- **FIFO:** Use the first in, first out (FIFO) method for storing groceries to prevent waste. When you bring home new groceries, make sure to move older items to the front of the pantry or fridge and put the newer items in the back. This way, you will eat the older items before they go bad and still be able to enjoy the new items after you have consumed the older ones. This means more healthy choices for a longer period of time.
- **List:** Keep a list of your Plan B food items on your fridge door (see Chapter 4 for the recommended list). When you use up one of the items, cross it out so you will remember to put it on your next grocery list. That way you will never be out of the ingredients you need to throw a healthy meal together in a snap.
- **Smart Storage:** Store items together by food group. For example, keep all your fruits and veggies on one shelf, meats and other proteins on one shelf, fats on one shelf, and whole grains/carbs together in the pantry. That way, when you are trying to quickly make a balanced meal according to our four-part meal pattern, you won't waste time looking for foods; you can simply grab an item from each group.

it's more important than ever to take a little extra time to be a mindful eater. So revisit the mindful-eating principles in Chapter 9 and try to eat sitting down, from a plate, and without distractions at least for a day or two until you feel like you're back in the swing of your healthy habits. At the very least, if you have to eat on the go, make sure your food is measured out so that you'll stop after a single serving without having to think twice.

When you don't have time to think twice about anything, you may want to stick to simple, whole foods rather than cooking up recipes. That will make it really easy to keep track of how well you are sticking to your meal pattern. A small sirloin steak, half a potato roasted in olive oil and rosemary, a sliced tomato, and steamed asparagus easily fit into the recommendations of the meal pattern. It will be easier to stick to a simple meal than trying to figure out more complex, combination foods like pizza or casseroles. Plus, these simple, whole foods tend to be naturally healthier and cleaner, which may help reset your taste buds and calm your cravings.

With the tools in this book, I think you will be pleasantly surprised how easy it is to get on track and stay on track. I'm excited for you because, perhaps for the first time, you'll be able to reach your goals without feeling stressed out or deprived of your favorite foods.

You'll watch with amazement as the pounds slip away—up to eight pounds in the first month! You'll feel energized not only from the weight loss but also from the fresh foods you're enjoying in the right portions at every meal. You'll feel better about how you look and feel.

Other things in your life will improve as well. You'll spend less money and time in the grocery store, all the while making smarter choices. You'll feel less stressed during the week since you'll have a plan, and even when that plan falls through you'll have a backup plan waiting in the wings.

In this life, instead of feeling stressed out and out of control, you will be able to navigate your busy schedule with ease, thanks to your weekly power-planning session. Instead of feeling run-down and chronically tired, you will feel energetic and motivated. Instead of eating whatever junk happens to be on hand when you get hungry, you'll be enjoying balanced meals and snacks that are easy to put together. This new life is empowering, fulfilling, and successful.

And the best part is that I know you can and will make this new life your own. If I can and my clients can, I know you can too. After a couple of weeks, you will see that 30 minutes a week is truly a small investment that gives a big return.

What you hold in your hand is a plan for success. Just 30 minutes of power planning each week will lead to weight loss, more energy, and less stress. Once you experience these results, you'll never want to miss a weekly planning session.

You're about to start a whole new life: a life in which food is no longer a source of guilt but rather a source of fuel and even pleasure. Energy will fill your life, and planning will free you from stress and from the drive-through! It will become second nature to spend a mere 30 minutes in power planning once a week, which will enable you to naturally keep the weight off and feel great forever!

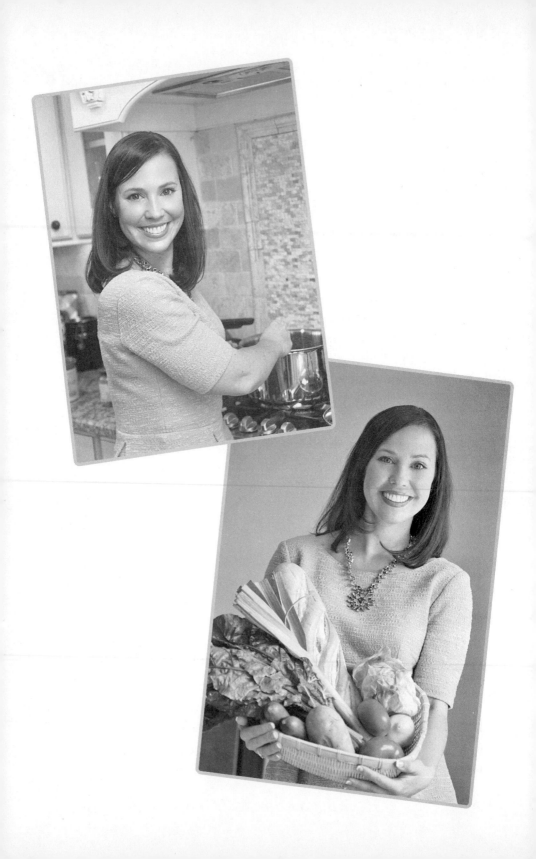

THE *SCHEDULE ME SKINNY* RECIPE COLLECTION

You've planned, you've shopped, you've prepped, and now it is time for the fun part—eating!! These recipes will provide you with a variety of healthy meals, snacks and treats to choose from that all fit within the suggested calorie ranges on the *Schedule Me Skinny* meal plan, making them easy to mix and match. I have included tips with several of the recipes.

I've also included the basic nutritional information for your reference. A few things to note: on many of the recipes I include the percent daily value (DV) for vitamins A and C, and minerals, calcium and iron, as these are the nutrients that appear on a standard nutrition facts panel. If the recipe contained one of these nutrients in an amount less than 5%, I considered that insignificant and therefore did not list the percent DV for those nutrients.

Remember: you don't have to count calories. If you are following the menu plans, the math has been done for you! The nutritional information here is to educate you and help you build your own menus going forward.

You'll enjoy a variety of meals using these recipes. Some take just minutes to make and others are perfect for times you want to make something a little more special. You'll never feel like you are on a diet when you get to enjoy these tasty meals!

Now, it's time to get cooking and chow down!

BREAKFASTS

Ooey-Gooey Strawberry Chocolate Chip Oatmeal

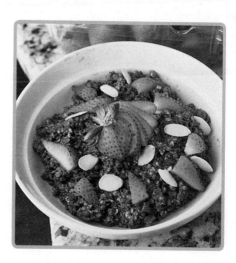

• • • • • •

ONE STUDY FOUND THAT DIETERS WHO ATE SWEETS FOR
BREAKFAST, ESPECIALLY CHOCOLATE, LOST MORE WEIGHT
THAN THOSE WHO DIDN'T, EVEN WHEN THEY ATE THE
SAME NUMBER OF CALORIES PER DAY!

2 packets unflavored instant
   oatmeal
1¾ cups skim milk
½ tbsp. honey
1 tsp. vanilla extract

¼ tsp. cinnamon
Pinch of nutmeg
2 tbsp. dark chocolate chips
1½ tbsp. sliced almonds, toasted
⅔ cup fresh strawberries, sliced

Prepare oatmeal according to package directions using milk.
While warm, stir in honey, vanilla extract, cinnamon, nutmeg, and
chocolate chips. Top with almonds and strawberries.

YIELD: 2 servings

NUTRITION FACTS PER SERVING: 360 calories, 9g fat, 3.5g sat fat, 115mg sodium, 56g
   carbs, 7g fiber, 14g protein, 8% DV vitamin A, 50% DV vitamin C, 25% DV
   calcium, 10% DV iron.

TOTAL PREPARATION TIME: 5 minutes

Peanut Butter and Berry Yogurt

● ● ● ● ● ●

THIS HEALTHY BREAKFAST IS LIKE A PORTABLE PB&J IN A CUP!

6 oz. nonfat vanilla Greek yogurt
1 tbsp. peanut butter
½ cup fresh berries

⇒ Mix yogurt and peanut butter thoroughly. Top with berries.

YIELD: 1 serving
NUTRITION FACTS PER SERVING: 230 calories, 8g fat, 1g sat fat, 125mg sodium, 23g carbs, 4g fiber, 15g protein, 20% DV vitamin C, 10% DV calcium.
TOTAL PREPARATION TIME: 3 minutes

Apple-Cinnamon Breakfast Pizza

• • • • • •

THIS IS ONE PIZZA YOU CAN FEEL GOOD ABOUT EATING FOR BREAKFAST! THE FIBER AND HEALTHY FATS WILL KEEP YOU FULL UNTIL LUNCH!

8-inch (80 calories) whole-wheat tortilla, such as La Tortilla Factory

1 tbsp. peanut butter
1 medium apple, thinly sliced
Cinnamon, to taste

Top the whole-wheat tortilla with the peanut butter, apple slices, and a sprinkle of cinnamon. To eat it on the go, just roll it up.

YIELD: 1 serving
NUTRITION FACTS PER SERVING: 270 calories, 10g fat, 1g sat fat, 300mg sodium, 40g carbs, 15g fiber, 7g protein, 8% DV vitamin C.
TOTAL PREPARATION TIME: 5 minutes

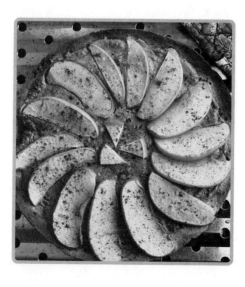

On-the-Go Omelet

· · · · · · ·

THIS IS AN OMELET YOU CAN TRULY EAT ON THE GO!

1 egg, beaten
2 tbsp. spinach or broccoli,
   chopped

2 tbsp. carrots, chopped
¼ cup shredded cheese
2 tbsp. salsa

Pour beaten egg into a small mug sprayed with cooking spray. Stir in spinach or broccoli, carrots, and cheese. Microwave mixture in the mug for 1 minute. Stir and then microwave for 30 seconds more or until egg is set. Serve with a dollop of salsa and enjoy on the go.

YIELD: 1 serving

NUTRITION FACTS PER SERVING: 130 calories, 8g fat, 3.5 sat fat, 350mg sodium, 5g carbs, 1g fiber, 10g protein, 60% DV vitamin A, 20% DV vitamin C, 15% DV calcium, 6% DV iron.

TOTAL PREPARATION TIME: 5 minutes

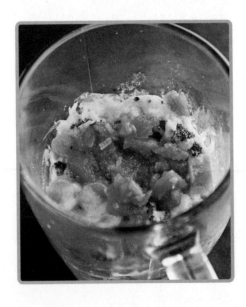

Peanut Butter and Banana Waffle Sandwich

• • • • • •

EATING THESE WAFFLES SANDWICH-STYLE MAKES THEM
EASY TO TAKE ON THE GO!

2 whole-grain frozen waffles
(such as Van's)
1 tbsp. peanut butter

1 banana, sliced
Cinnamon, to taste

⇒ Toast waffles according to package directions. Spread one waffle
with peanut butter and top with banana slices. Top with the other
waffle and eat!

YIELD: 1 serving
NUTRITION FACTS PER SERVING: 360 calories, 8g fat, 1g sat fat, 730mg sodium, 49g
carbs, 8g fiber, 12g protein, 8% DV vitamin C, 35% DV calcium, 40% DV iron.
TOTAL PREPARATION TIME: 5 minutes

Berry Granola Parfait

· · · · · ·

GREEK YOGURT MAKES THIS A PROTEIN-PACKED BREAK-
FAST AND THE HONEY ADDS A SWEET FLAVOR!

6 oz. plain nonfat Greek yogurt
1 cup fresh berries (blueberries
   and raspberries work well)

¼ cup granola
1 tbsp. honey

▷ Layer first three ingredients in a glass, parfait-style. Drizzle with
honey and enjoy on the go!

· ·

YIELD: 1 serving
NUTRITION FACTS PER SERVING: 340 calories, 3g fat, 0g sat fat, 125mg sodium, 60g
   carbs, 7g fiber, 23g protein, 50% DV vitamin C, 20% DV calcium, 6% DV iron.
TOTAL PREPARATION TIME: 3 minutes

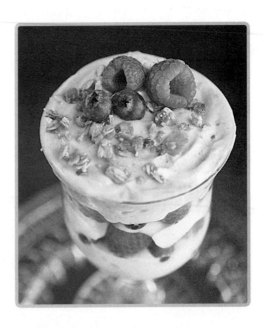

Easy Egg Fiesta Wrap

• • • • • • •

THIS WRAP COMBINES HEALTHY FATS, VEGGIES,
AND PROTEIN FOR AN ON-THE-GO BREAKFAST WITH
STAYING POWER!

1 large egg, beaten
1 100% whole-wheat tortilla
   (pick one that has 150 calories
   or less)

½ cup chopped spinach
2 tbsp. salsa
¼ cup shredded cheese

Pour beaten egg in a small bowl sprayed with cooking spray. Microwave in 30-second intervals until cooked through. Top tortilla with cooked egg, spinach, salsa, and cheese.

YIELD: 1 serving
NUTRITION FACTS PER SERVING: 230 calories, 11g fat, 6g sat fat, 660mg sodium, 16g carbs, 9g fiber, 14g protein, 15% DV vitamin A, 20% DV calcium.
TOTAL PREPARATION TIME: 5 minutes

Peanut Butter Banana Flax Oatmeal

• • • • • •

BANANA, BROWN SUGAR, AND PEANUT BUTTER UP THE "YUM" FACTOR OF THIS OATMEAL WHILE THE GROUND FLAXSEED ADDS HEALTHY OMEGA-3 FATS AND FIBER!

1 packet unflavored instant oatmeal

1 medium banana, mashed

1 tbsp. peanut butter

1 tbsp. ground flaxseed

1 tsp. brown sugar

⇝ Cook oatmeal in microwave according to package directions. Once cooked, stir in mashed banana and peanut butter. Top with ground flaxseed and brown sugar.

YIELD: 1 serving

NUTRITION FACTS PER SERVING: 360 calories, 13g fat, 1.5g sat fat, 165mg sodium, 54g carbs, 10g fiber, 12.5g protein, 8% DV vitamin A, 8% DV vitamin C, 20% DV calcium, 10% DV iron.

TOTAL PREPARATION TIME: 5 minutes

LUNCHES

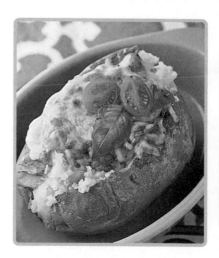

Italian-Style Loaded Potato

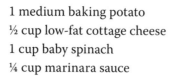

ALL THE FLAVORS OF A PIZZA COME TOGETHER IN THIS SUPER-QUICK SPUD!

1 medium baking potato
½ cup low-fat cottage cheese
1 cup baby spinach
¼ cup marinara sauce

1 tbsp. mozzarella cheese
Italian herb blend (or a sprinkle each of dried oregano and basil)

Pierce potato several times with a fork. Microwave for 4 minutes. Meanwhile, stir together cottage cheese, baby spinach, and marinara sauce. Slice the potato open, stuff with cottage cheese mixture, and sprinkle with cheese and a dash of Italian herb blend. Then microwave 1 minute more until heated through.

YIELD: 1 serving
NUTRITION FACTS PER SERVING: 300 calories, 3.5g fat, 2g sat fat, 770mg sodium, 50g carbs, 6g fiber, 20g protein, 25% DV vitamin A, 45% DV vitamin C, 30% DV calcium, 20% DV iron.
TOTAL PREPARATION TIME: 6 minutes

Salmon and Chickpea Lettuce Wraps

• • • • • •

ASIAN LETTUCE WRAPS ARE POPULAR, BUT THESE
LETTUCE WRAPS OFFER A FRESH TWIST WITH
MEDITERRANEAN FLAVORS!

1 (3 oz.) can salmon
½ cup canned chickpeas, rinsed
   and drained
1 tbsp. extra-virgin olive oil
2 tsp. lemon juice

1 tbsp. sun-dried tomatoes,
   chopped
Dried dill
6 Bibb lettuce leaves

➢ Drain salmon and toss with chickpeas, olive oil, lemon juice, sun-dried tomatoes, and a sprinkle of dried dill. Serve in Bibb lettuce leaves.

YIELD: 1 serving

NUTRITION FACTS PER SERVING: 360 calories, 19g fat, 2.5g sat fat, 610mg sodium, 21g carbs, 5g fiber, 27g protein, 35% DV vitamin A, 10% DV vitamin C, 10% DV calcium, 15% DV iron.

TOTAL PREPARATION TIME: 5 minutes

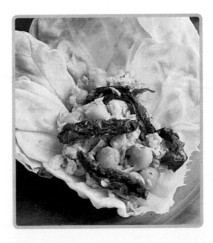

Lentil-Stuffed Peppers

● ● ● ● ● ●

IF YOU CAN'T FIND CANNED LENTILS IN YOUR GROCERY
STORE, BUY REDUCED-SODIUM LENTIL SOUP AND DRAIN THE
LIQUID SO THAT YOU ARE LEFT WITH JUST THE LENTILS.

1 large bell pepper
½ cup canned lentils, rinsed
  and drained

½ cup salsa
¼ cup shredded cheese

Cut bell pepper in half lengthwise and remove insides and seeds.
Microwave on high 2 minutes to soften. Set aside. Combine lentils
and salsa, then fill each bell pepper half with half of the mixture.
Microwave another 2 minutes or until warmed through. Sprinkle
each half evenly with cheese and microwave another 30 seconds or
so until the cheese melts.

YIELD: 1 serving
NUTRITION FACTS PER SERVING: 260 calories, 6g fat, 3.5g sat fat, 840mg sodium, 33g
  carbs, 11g fiber, 17g protein, 100% DV vitamin A, 330% DV vitamin C, 35% DV
  calcium, 10% DV iron.
TOTAL PREPARATION TIME: 6 minutes

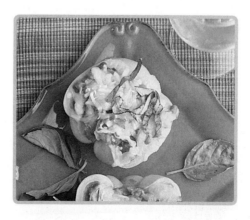

Nutty Quinoa Salad with Strawberries

• • • • • •

USE LEFTOVER QUINOA AND THIS NUTTY SALAD WILL
COME TOGETHER IN SECONDS!

½ cup cooked quinoa (¼ cup dry)
½ cup sliced strawberries
1 cup spinach
2 tbsp. sliced almonds

1 oz. crumbled goat or Feta
cheese
Basil leaves (optional)

Toss together first five ingredients. Top with a few torn basil
leaves if desired.

YIELD: 1 serving

NUTRITION FACTS PER SERVING: 330 calories, 18g fat, 7g sat fat, 190mg sodium, 32g
carbs, 7g fiber, 15g protein, 25% DV vitamin A, 80% DV vitamin C, 15% DV
calcium, 20% DV iron.

TOTAL PREPARATION TIME: 5 minutes

Tuna, Lettuce, and Tomato

● ● ● ● ● ●

GREEK YOGURT CUTS THE FAT, WHILE KEEPING THE FLAVOR OF THIS LUNCHTIME FAVORITE!

1 (5 oz.) can of tuna, drained
1 tbsp. light mayonnaise (such as canola oil mayo)
3 tbsp. nonfat Greek yogurt
Salt and pepper, to taste

2 slices 100% whole-wheat bread
1–2 Bibb lettuce leaves or a handful of spinach
2 tomato slices

▷ Combine first three ingredients, mixing well. Season with salt and pepper to taste. Spread mixture on one slice of 100% whole-wheat bread. Top with a piece of lettuce or spinach and two tomato slices, then the other slice of bread.

YIELD: 1 serving
NUTRITION FACTS PER SERVING: 430 calories, 14g fat, 1.5g sat fat, 450mg sodium, 30g carbs, 5g fiber, 45g protein, 25% DV vitamin A, 20% DV vitamin C, 15% DV calcium, 20% DV iron.
TOTAL PREPARATION TIME: 5 minutes

DINNERS

Portabella Pizzas

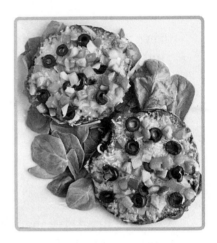

YES, YOU CAN EAT TWO WHOLE
PIZZAS FOR DINNER AND STILL
LOSE WEIGHT!

2 large portabella caps
4 tbsp. marinara sauce
¼ cup shredded mozzarella
   cheese

Veggie toppings of your choice,
   such as peppers and olives
Italian herb blend (or a sprinkle
   each of dried oregano and basil)
   (optional)

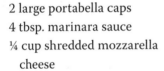 Preheat oven to 350°F. Top each portabella half evenly with marinara sauce, cheese, and veggies. Sprinkle with Italian seasoning, if desired. Bake until warmed through and cheese has melted (about 10 minutes). Alternatively, you can microwave 1–2 minutes.

YIELD: 1 serving

NUTRITION FACTS PER SERVING: 220 calories, 10g fat, 3.5g sat fat, 620mg sodium, 18g carbs, 5g fiber, 15g protein, 30% DV vitamin A, 90% DV vitamin C, 30% DV calcium, 15% DV iron.

TOTAL PREPARATION TIME: 15 minutes for oven method or 5 minutes for microwave method

DINNERS

Mini Meat Loaves

● ● ● ● ● ●

USE A MUFFIN TIN TO MAKE THESE MEAT LOAVES
A SUPER-CUTE MINI-SIZE AND PROVIDE BUILT-IN
PORTION CONTROL!

1 lb. lean ground beef
1/3 cup oatmeal (can use from
   instant packet)
1 egg, beaten
½ cup chopped onion

¼ tsp. each salt and pepper
2 tbsp. marinara sauce
Large dash of Worcestershire
   sauce

Preheat oven to 375°F. In a large bowl, mix lean ground beef with oatmeal, beaten egg, chopped onion, salt and pepper, marinara sauce, and Worcestershire sauce. Using an ice cream scoop, divide the mixture in a 12-cup muffin tin that has been sprayed with cooking spray. Bake for 25 minutes or until cooked through. Drizzle each meat loaf with an additional tablespoon of marinara sauce just before serving.

YIELD: 6 servings

NUTRITION FACTS PER SERVING: 110 calories, 3.5g fat, 1.5g sat fat, 160mg sodium, 5g carbs, 1g fiber, 16g protein, 8% DV iron.

TOTAL PREPARATION TIME: 35 minutes

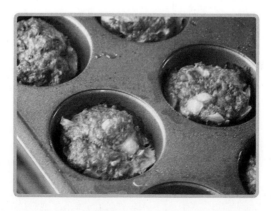

Roast Beef Melt

● ● ● ● ● ●

**THE VEGGIES HELP CREATE A HEALTHY TWIST ON
THIS CLASSIC SATISFYING SAMMY.**

4 slices 100% whole-wheat bread
6 oz. roast beef
2 tsp. olive oil
1 cup sliced mushrooms
1 cup sliced yellow onion
½ cup mozzarella cheese

Freshly ground black pepper,
    to taste
1 cup arugula or 4 Bibb lettuce
    leaves
Mustard (optional)

*NOTE: *The first step is optional: To save time, skip the sauté and top the
sandwich with raw onion and mushrooms.*

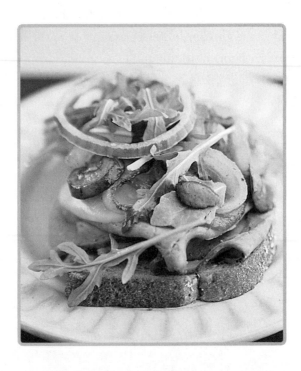

⇢ Heat olive oil in a nonstick skillet over medium-high heat. Add mushrooms and yellow onions and sauté until softened and onion turns slightly golden brown. Remove from heat and set aside.

Evenly divide the roast beef, the sautéed (or raw) mushrooms and onions, and cheese on two slices of the bread. Optional: Toast under broiler until cheese melts. Then sprinkle each half generously with fresh black pepper and finish by topping with arugula or lettuce, mustard, if desired, and other slices of bread.

YIELD: 2 servings

NUTRITION FACTS PER SERVING: 440 calories, 13g fat, 4.5g sat fat, 920mg sodium, 44g carbs, 6g fiber, 38g protein, 8% DV vitamin A, 15% DV vitamin C, 35% DV calcium, 25% DV iron.

TOTAL PREPARATION TIME: 15 minutes with the sauté method or 5 minutes using raw onions and mushrooms

Pan-Glazed Chicken with Kale and Basil

● ● ● ● ● ●

THE SWEETNESS FROM THE BALSAMIC VINEGAR
AND HONEY STAND UP TO THE BITTER FLAVORS OF
THE FRESH KALE, MAKING FOR A TRULY SWEET
AND SAVORY EXPERIENCE.

4 (4 oz.) chicken breasts, skinned
  and boned
½ tsp. salt
½ tsp. fresh ground pepper
2 tsp. olive oil
2 tbsp. balsamic vinegar

2 tbsp. honey
2–3 cups chopped fresh kale
2 tbsp. chopped fresh basil
  (optional)
1 tbsp. crumbled goat cheese

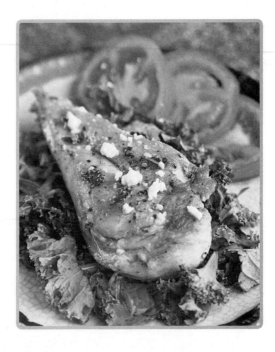

⤳ Sprinkle both sides of chicken with salt and pepper. Heat oil in a large nonstick or iron skillet over medium-high heat. Add chicken and cook 5 minutes or until lightly browned. Turn chicken and cook 6 minutes or until chicken is done. Stir in vinegar, honey, and kale and cook just until kale is wilted. Remove from heat; sprinkle with goat cheese and basil just before serving.

YIELD: 4 servings

NUTRITION FACTS PER SERVING: 216 calories, 14g carbs, 25g protein, 6g fat, 1g sat fat, 460mg sodium, 1g fiber, 130% DV vitamin A, 87% DV vitamin C, 8% DV calcium, 7% DV iron.

TOTAL PREPARATION TIME: 15 minutes

DINNERS

Sarah-Jane and Joe's Blackened Salmon

• • • • • •

MY HUBBY AND I CREATED THIS RECIPE ONE BUSY WEEK-
NIGHT, AND NOW IT IS OUR WEEKLY GO-TO DINNER.

2 tsp. blackened seasoning
2 tsp. Old Bay seasoning
2 tsp. dark brown sugar

2 tbsp. olive oil, divided
4 (4 oz.) salmon fillets, skin
   removed

⟫ Combine the blackened seasoning, Old Bay seasoning, and dark brown sugar in a small bowl. Set aside. Drizzle 1 tbsp. of olive oil evenly over the salmon fillets and rub in. Then rub the fillets evenly on both sides with the seasoning mixture. Heat the other tablespoon of olive oil in a nonstick skillet (we actually love to use our cast-iron skillet) over medium-high heat. Add the salmon and cook for 5–6 minutes on each side or until done.

YIELD: 4 servings
NUTRITION FACTS PER SERVING: 230 calories, 14g fat, 2g sat fat, 600mg sodium, 2g
   carbs, 0g fiber, 23g protein, 6% DV iron.
TOTAL PREPARATION TIME: 15 minutes

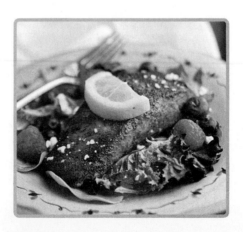

Mediterranean Quinoa Bowl

• • • • • •

THIS SIMPLE SUPPER COMBINES WONDERFUL SAVORY
MEDITERRANEAN FLAVORS WITH STAYING POWER FROM
PROTEIN POWERHOUSES FISH AND QUINOA.

4 tbsp. extra-virgin olive oil
2 tbsp. red wine or balsamic
   vinegar
1 tsp. Dijon mustard
Salt and pepper to taste
8 cups baby spinach
2 cups cooked quinoa
12 oz. canned salmon or tuna,
   drained

6–7 oz. crumbled Feta
1 cup artichoke hearts (optional)
1 cup tomatoes, diced
1 cup cucumbers, diced
½ cup Kalamata olives, sliced
   (optional)

Whisk together the first three ingredients and season with salt
and pepper to make the dressing. Set aside. In a large bowl, layer the
baby spinach, quinoa, salmon or tuna, Feta, artichoke hearts (if
desired), tomatoes, cucumbers, and olives (if desired). Serve with
dressing on the side. Enjoy!

YIELD: 4 servings

NUTRITION FACTS PER SERVING: 430 calories, 21g fat, 5g sat fat, 800mg sodium, 31g
   carbs, 6g fiber, 30g protein, 45% DV vitamin A, 25% DV vitamin C, 20% DV
   calcium, 35% DV iron.

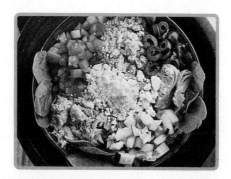

Black Jack Tacos

• • • • • •

THIS EASY DISH CAN BE MADE IN MINUTES JUST USING
THE MICROWAVE! TO KEEP THE SALT CONTENT FROM BEING
TOO HIGH, BE SURE TO RINSE AND DRAIN THE CANNED
BEANS, WHICH WILL REDUCE THE SODIUM BY 40%.

2 whole-wheat tortillas (such as
La Tortilla Factory Smart &
Delicious Whole-Wheat
Tortillas)

½ cup canned black beans, rinsed
and drained

4 tbsp. shredded cheese

2 tbsp. homemade or store-
bought salsa (either a spicy
tomato salsa or a cool pineapple
salsa works great)

2 tbsp. cumin cream (see recipe
below)

Shredded lettuce or cabbage
(optional)

Cilantro leaves (optional)

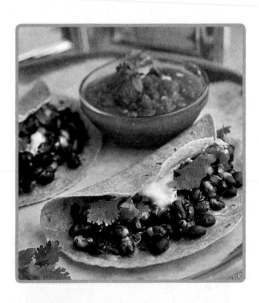

⤳ Top each tortilla with ¼ cup beans and 2 tbsp. cheese. Heat, if desired, in the microwave for 1 minute on high or until the tortilla and beans are warm and the cheese is melted.

Remove and top each taco with 1 tbsp. salsa and 1 tbsp. cumin cream. Finish by topping each taco with shredded lettuce or cabbage and cilantro leaves.

YIELD: 1 serving
NUTRITION FACTS PER SERVING (2 TACOS): 300 calories, 6g fat, 1.5g sat fat, 356mg sodium, 48g carbs, 9g fiber, 15g protein, 30% DV calcium, 40% DV Vitamin C, 8% DV vitamin A, 20% DV iron.

Cumin Cream

¼ cup nonfat plain Greek yogurt
½ tsp. cumin
1 tsp. lime or lemon juice

⤳ Whisk all ingredients together in a small bowl until smooth and mixed thoroughly. Season with salt and pepper, if desired.

NOTE: Leftover cumin cream can be refrigerated for 3–4 days and makes a great dip for raw veggies.
NUTRITION FACTS PER SERVING (2 TBSP.): 10 calories, 0g fat, 0g sat fat, 25mg sodium, 1g carbs, 1g protein, 0g fiber.
TOTAL PREPARATION TIME FOR TACOS AND CUMIN CREAM: 8 minutes

No-Mess Baked Fish and Veggies

••••••

MILD WHITE FISH, LIKE TILAPIA, IS ONE OF THE LOWEST-CALORIE SOURCES OF PROTEIN. THE GOOD NEWS IS THAT IT'S INEXPENSIVE TOO! THIS FISH DINNER IS COOKED IN A PACKET WITH THE VEGGIES TO KEEP ALL THE GREAT FLAVOR AND MOISTURE IN! FROZEN MIXED VEGGIES ARE A NUTRITIONAL BARGAIN: PAY JUST A QUARTER FOR A 1-CUP SERVING THAT PROVIDES 6G FIBER AND A WHOPPING 115% OF YOUR DAILY VALUE FOR VITAMIN A!

4 (6 oz.) tilapia fillets

2 tsp. Old Bay Seasoning

4 cups frozen mixed vegetables
   (1 cup per fillet)

Salt and pepper to taste

2 tsp. dried thyme (½ tsp. for each
   fillet)

8 tsp. olive oil (2 tsp. per fillet)

4 tsp. white wine, water, broth
   (1 tsp. for each fillet)

4 lemon slices

2 cups cooked quinoa (for
   serving)

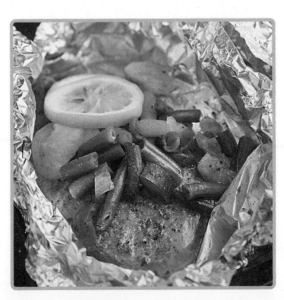

Preheat oven to 400°F. Place each tilapia fillet in the center of a large piece (12″ by 18″) of aluminum foil and sprinkle with Old Bay seasoning. Top the fillet with 1 cup frozen mixed vegetables and sprinkle with salt, pepper, and thyme. Drizzle with olive oil and wine and top with a lemon slice. Roll foil up to secure each packet for baking. Bake for 25 minutes or until fish flakes easily with a fork and veggies are crisp-tender. Serve with ½ cup quinoa per person.

YIELD: 4 servings

NUTRITION FACTS PER SERVING: 450 calories, 13g fat, 2.5g sat fat, 920mg sodium, 42g carbs, 5g fiber, 40g protein, 45% DV vitamin A, 10% DV vitamin C, 6% DV calcium, 15% DV iron.

TOTAL PREPARATION TIME: 30 minutes

DINNERS

SLOW-COOKER DINNERS

Slow-Cooker Pulled Pork Tacos

• • • • • •

THESE PORK TACOS WILL WOW YOU WITH THEIR TENDER
TEXTURE AND SWEET-HEAT FLAVOR!

1 lb. extra-lean pork tenderloin
½ tsp. Mrs. Dash Southwest
   Chipotle Seasoning
½ tsp. salt
¼ tsp. pepper
1 onion, chopped
¾ cup premade red enchilada
   sauce
½ cup light beer
½ cup barbecue sauce
2 tbsp. hot sauce (such as Texas
   Pete)
12 whole-wheat tortillas
1 cup shredded cabbage

⇨ Place pork tenderloin in a slow-cooker that has been sprayed with cooking spray. Sprinkle chipotle seasoning, salt, and pepper directly onto the pork. Add onion, red enchilada sauce, light beer, barbecue sauce and hot sauce. Cook, covered, on low for 8 hours. After cooking, shred pork with a fork and serve with the sauce from the pot on tortillas, with cabbage and any other toppings of your choice.

YIELD: 6 servings, 2 tacos per serving
NUTRITION FACTS PER SERVING: 270 calories, 3.5g fat, 0.5g sat fat, 750mg sodium,
   39g carbs, 5g fiber, 19g protein, 45% DV vitamin C, 8% DV iron.
TOTAL PREPARATION TIME: 15 minutes plus 8 hours cook time

Slow-Cooker Sweet Potatoes

● ● ● ● ● ●

SERVE THESE WITH THE PAN-GLAZED CHICKEN
FOR A COLORFUL, EASY DINNER.

7 cups sweet potatoes, chopped
  into chunks
1 yellow onion, coarsely chopped
2 tbsp. olive oil

2 tsp. dried dill weed
1 tsp. brown sugar
½ tsp. salt
½ tsp. pepper

Toss all ingredients in a bowl until well combined. Place in slow-cooker that has been sprayed with cooking spray. Cook on low for 4½ hours.

YIELD: 4 servings

NUTRITION FACTS PER SERVING: 200 calories, 7g fat, 1g sat fat, 360mg sodium, 31g carbs, 5g fiber, 3g protein, 370% DV vitamin A, 10% DV vitamin C, 6% DV calcium, 6% DV iron.

TOTAL PREPARATION TIME: 10 minutes plus 4½ hours cook time

DINNERS

Slow-Cooker Mediterranean Chicken

• • • • • •

4 (4 oz.) boneless, skinless
    chicken breasts
3 tbsp. olive oil
2 tbsp. balsamic vinegar
½ cup lower-sodium chicken
    broth
1 tsp. minced garlic
¼ cup chopped fresh oregano
    (or 2 tbsp. dried oregano)

1 tsp. dried rosemary
2 tsp. dried thyme
¼ tsp. salt
½ tsp. freshly ground black
    pepper
Fresh basil (optional)

▷ Brush chicken breasts with olive oil and place in a slow-cooker that has been sprayed with cooking spray. Combine the rest of the ingredients except basil and pour mixture over chicken. Cover and cook on low for 5 hours until cooked through. Serve topped with a spoonful of the sauce from the Crock-Pot and sprinkle with fresh basil, over a bed of couscous or on top of a salad.

YIELD: 4 servings
NUTRITION FACTS PER SERVING: 210 calories, 10g fat, 1g sat fat, 560mg sodium, 3g
    carbs, 0g fiber, 27g protein, 8% DV iron.
TOTAL PREPARATION TIME: 5 minutes plus 5 hours cook time

PLAN B DINNERS

Vegetable Burger with Sweet Potato Fries

• • • • • • •

THIS BURGER-AND-FRIES COMBO WILL SATISFY
YOUR CRAVINGS AND BE READY FASTER THAN THE
DRIVE-THROUGH!

½ large sweet potato
1 tbsp. olive oil
Salt and pepper, to taste
1 frozen veggie burger (such as
    MorningStar Farms' Chipotle
    Black Bean)

1 whole-wheat sandwich thin
Ketchup
Mustard

Peel the sweet potato and cut into strips. Drizzle with olive oil, salt, and pepper. Toss well and lay on a baking sheet. Bake at 425°F for 20 minutes or until crispy. While fries are baking, cook burger according to package directions. Toast sandwich thin. Assemble burger with your choice of toppings.

YIELD: 1 serving.

NUTRITION FACTS PER SERVING: 450 calories, 22g fat, 3g sat fat, 510 mg sodium, 45g carbs, 8g fiber, 20g protein, 350% DV vitamin A, 30% DV vitamin C, 8% DV calcium, 20% DV iron.

TOTAL PREPARATION TIME: 30 minutes

DINNERS

Tuna Edamame Wraps

• • • • • •

THESE EASY-TO-MAKE WRAPS ARE LOADED WITH SPICY
FLAVOR AND FILLING PROTEIN AND FIBER.

1 cup diced frozen red onion
½ cup cooked-from-frozen shelled
  edamame
1 (5 oz.) can chunk light tuna
  packed in water, drained
½ cup canned chickpeas, rinsed
  and drained
¼ tsp. Sriracha hot sauce
Salt and pepper to taste
2 tbsp. salsa
¾ cup frozen chopped spinach,
  cooked
2 corn tortillas

▷ Heat onions in microwave for 30 seconds or until thawed. In a mixing bowl, combine all ingredients except spinach and corn tortillas. Arrange half the spinach in the center of each tortilla. Spread tuna and edamame mixture evenly on each tortilla, add remaining spinach on top of each tortilla, and wrap each one tightly. Cut each wrap in half and serve with 1 cup cooked frozen mixed veggies per person.

YIELD: 2 servings
NUTRITION FACTS PER SERVING: 450 calories, 4g fat, 0g sat fat, 420 mg sodium, 60g
  carbohydrates, 12g fiber, 35g protein, 150% DV vitamin A, 20% DV vitamin C,
  12% DV calcium, 20% DV iron.
TOTAL PREPARATION TIME: 15 minutes

Pasta with Sautéed Spinach, Toasted Pine Nuts, and Chicken

· · · · · ·

THIS PASTA PROVIDES EVERYTHING YOU LOVE ABOUT
COMFORT FOOD FOR FEWER CALORIES!

½ cup whole-wheat pasta

1 tbsp. pine nuts

1½ tbsp. olive oil

½ cup frozen diced yellow onion

1 tsp. minced garlic

2 tbsp. seasoned sun-dried
tomatoes (such as Bella Sun
Luci with Greek oregano, basil,
and garlic)

1 (6 oz.) can diced chicken breast

1½ cup spinach, thawed

¼ tsp. salt

¼ tsp. pepper to taste

2 tsp. Parmesan (optional)

Cook the pasta al dente according to package directions. While pasta is cooking, heat a large skillet over low heat. Add pine nuts and toast until golden brown. (Watch carefully, as they brown fairly quickly.) Remove nuts from pan and set aside. Heat olive oil in the skillet. Add onion, garlic, sun-dried tomatoes, and chicken to the skillet and cook until the onion begins to soften and chicken is warmed through, about 5–7 minutes. Drain pasta and add it to the skillet. Squeeze spinach to remove excess water and add it to the skillet. Stir until the spinach begins to soften. Toss in the pine nuts and add salt and pepper to taste. Sprinkle with cheese, if desired, and serve.

YIELD: 2 servings

NUTRITION FACTS PER SERVING: 450 calories, 22g fat, 4.5g sat fat, 890mg sodium, 25g carbs, 5g fiber, 33g protein, 120% DV vitamin A, 15% DV vitamin C, 25% DV calcium, 20% DV iron.

TOTAL PREPARATION TIME: 15 minutes

DINNERS

Chipotle Grilled Salmon with Pineapple Salsa and Quinoa

● ● ● ● ● ●

THE CHIPOTLE AND PINEAPPLE SALSA GIVE THIS SALMON
SUCH GREAT FLAVOR, YOU'LL WANT TO MAKE IT AGAIN
AND AGAIN!

½ cup frozen diced red onion

1 (15 oz.) can pineapple tidbits in
100% juice, drained

½ tsp. dried basil (optional)

2 tsp. honey

1 tsp. Mrs. Dash Southwest
Chipotle seasoning

½ tsp. brown sugar

½ tsp. cumin

Salt and pepper to taste

4 (5 oz.) fillets frozen salmon that
can be cooked from frozen,
such as Gorton's Classic
Grilled Salmon

2 cups cooked quinoa (1 cup dry)

6 cups frozen steam-in-the-bag
mixed vegetables

Heat the frozen onion in a nonstick skillet just until thawed.
Combine all the salsa ingredients (red onion, pineapple, dried basil,
and honey) in a medium bowl. Refrigerate until ready to use. In a
small bowl, combine chipotle seasoning, brown sugar, cumin, salt,
and pepper. Rub salmon piece well with spice mixture. Cook salmon
according to package directions. While salmon is cooking, prepare
quinoa according to package directions and heat vegetables according
to package directions. Spoon ½ cup quinoa on each of 4 plates, place
a salmon fillet on top of the quinoa on each plate, and top with salsa
mixture. Serve with 1½ cups cooked frozen mixed veggies per person.

YIELD: 4 servings

NUTRITION FACTS PER SERVING: 440 calories, 5g fat, 0.5g sat fat, 340mg sodium, 60g
carbs, 9g fiber, 25g protein, 200% DV vitamin A, 15% DV vitamin C, 14% DV iron.

TOTAL PREPARATION TIME: 20 minutes

DINNERS

Chicken and Vegetable Quinoa

• • • • • •

CREATE A FULL, BALANCED MEAL IN 20 MINUTES
WITH THIS RECIPE!

2 tbsp. olive oil

2 cloves garlic, minced

1 (3 oz.) can diced chicken breast, drained

1½ cups frozen mixed vegetables

½ cup cooked quinoa (¼ cup dry)

¼ cup canned chickpeas, rinsed and drained

Salt and pepper to taste

Heat olive oil and garlic in a large sauté skillet. Add chicken and cook until it is warmed through, about a minute. Add frozen vegetables and cook for another 5–7 minutes. Meanwhile, reheat quinoa in the microwave. Add chickpeas to chicken and vegetable mixture and stir. Add cooked and warmed quinoa to chicken and vegetable mixture and remove from heat. Stir until all ingredients are well incorporated. Add salt and pepper to taste.

YIELD: 2 servings

NUTRITION FACTS PER SERVING: 460 calories, 18g fat, 3g sat fat, 210mg sodium, 55g carbs, 5g fiber, 19g protein, 35% DV vitamin A, 10% DV vitamin C, 6% DV calcium, 10% DV iron.

TOTAL PREPARATION TIME: 20 minutes

DINNERS

Black Bean Soup with Baked Tortilla Chips

THIS SOUP IS FILLING WITHOUT LEAVING YOU FEELING TOO FULL. SERVE WITH BAKED TORTILLA CHIPS TO ADD THE PERFECT CRUNCH.

1 tbsp. olive oil
1 cup diced frozen red onion
4 cloves garlic, chopped
1 tbsp. chili powder
1 tbsp. cumin
½ tbsp. smoked paprika
3 cups lower-sodium chicken broth

3 (15 oz.) cans lower-sodium black beans
3 (15 oz.) cans whole kernel corn
1 (14½ oz.) can crushed tomatoes
8 oz. baked tortilla chips
10 cups pineapple tidbits in juice

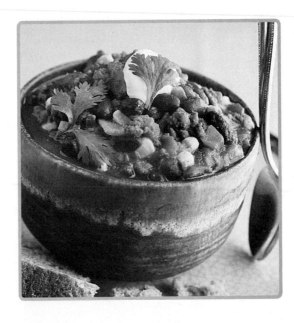

▷ Heat oil in a large saucepan over medium heat. Add onion and garlic and cook and stir until they begin to soften. Add chili powder, cumin, and smoked paprika; then cook and stir for 1 minute. Add broth, beans, corn, and tomatoes. Bring to a boil; then reduce heat and simmer for 10 minutes. Remove from heat and serve with 1 oz. baked tortilla chips and 1¼ cups canned pineapple tidbits in juice per person.

. . . .

YIELD: 8 servings

NUTRITION FACTS PER SERVING: 440 calories, 3g fat, 0g sat fat, 950mg sodium, 85g carbs, 15g fiber, 10g protein, 6% DV vitamin A, 80% DV vitamin C, 8% DV calcium, 25% DV iron.

TOTAL PREPARATION TIME: 20 minutes

SNACKS

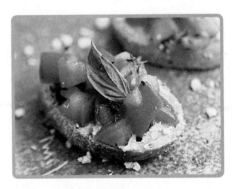

Sarah-Jane's Goat Cheese Bruschetta

• • • • • •

THIS IS A GREAT SNACK TO SERVE AS AN APPETIZER TO
DINNER GUESTS. IT'S EASY TO MAKE, COMES TOGETHER IN
MINUTES, AND IS ALWAYS A CROWD-PLEASER.

1 cup chopped heirloom tomatoes
2 tsp. chopped fresh oregano or
  1 tsp. dried oregano
1 tsp. chopped thyme or ½ tsp.
  dried thyme
1 tbsp. extra-virgin olive oil
2 tsp. balsamic vinegar
¼ tsp. salt

⅛ tsp. freshly ground black
  pepper
6 oz. soft goat cheese
6 small slices crusty whole-grain
  bread
6 fresh basil leaves, sliced
(optional)

Combine first 7 ingredients in a medium bowl, tossing gently. Let stand 10 minutes. Spread goat cheese evenly on each bread slice. Spread a spoonful of bruschetta onto each slice of bread on top of the cheese. Sprinkle each piece with sliced basil, if desired. Serve immediately.

YIELD: 6 servings
NUTRITION FACTS PER SERVING: 200 calories, 12g fat, 6g sat fat, 340mg sodium, 13g carbs, 2g fiber, 10g protein, 10% DV vitamin A, 10% DV calcium, 8% DV iron.
TOTAL PREPARATION TIME: 20 minutes

Nutty Choco Popcorn

······

**SALTY, SAVORY, AND SWEET—THIS SNACK IS
THE PERFECT CURE FOR ANY CRAVING!**

2 tbsp. popcorn kernels
2 tbsp. dry-roasted almonds
1 tbsp. dark chocolate chips
Salt to taste

Place popcorn kernels into a lunch-size brown paper bag and fold over several times. Microwave on high for 1 to 1½ minutes or until the popping slows. Toss popcorn with almonds, chocolate chips, and salt.

YIELD: 1 serving
NUTRITION FACTS PER SERVING: 210 calories, 13g fat, 3.5g sat fat, 0mg sodium, 20g carbs, 4g fiber, 6g protein, 6% DV iron.
TOTAL PREPARATION TIME: 3 minutes

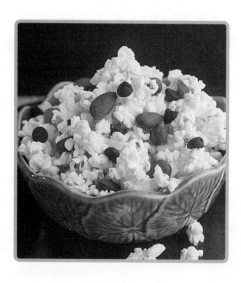

SNACKS

Loaded Banana

● ● ● ● ● ●

THIS IS A HEALTHIER VERSION OF A TREAT-ON-A-STICK
LIKE YOU GET AT THE SUMMER FAIR!

½ medium banana, peeled
1 tbsp. peanut butter
2 tbsp. crushed granola or sliced
  almonds
2 tsp. raisins

Spread peanut butter evenly on banana. Toss crushed cereal or almonds and raisins together in a small bowl. Roll banana in cereal-and-raisin mixture.

YIELD: 1 serving
NUTRITION FACTS PER SERVING: 190 calories, 9g fat, 0.5g sat fat, 65mg sodium, 25g carbs, 4g fiber, 4g protein, 15% DV vitamin C, 8% DV calcium, 10% DV iron.
TOTAL PREPARATION TIME: 3 minutes

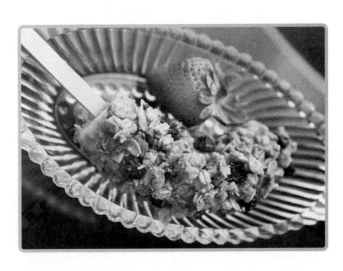

SNACKS

Angel Eggs

● ● ● ● ● ● ●

I CALL THESE "ANGEL EGGS" BECAUSE UNLIKE
THE DISH THAT INSPIRED THEM, THERE'S NOTHING
DEVILISH ABOUT THEM!

1 hard-boiled egg, peeled	Salt and pepper to taste
1 tbsp. hummus	Smoked paprika (optional)
1 tbsp. plain nonfat Greek yogurt	

➢ Slice egg in half lengthwise. Remove yolk and place in a small
bowl with hummus and Greek yogurt. Add salt and pepper to taste.
Mix thoroughly and then spoon into each egg half. Sprinkle with
smoked paprika, if desired.

YIELD: 1 serving
NUTRITION FACTS PER SERVING: 90 calories, 5g fat, 1g sat fat, 115mg sodium, 4g
carbs, 1g fiber, 8g protein.
TOTAL PREPARATION TIME: 5 minutes

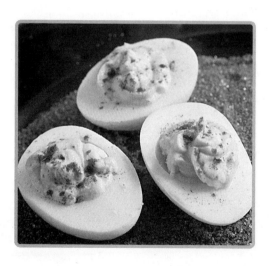

SNACKS

TREATS

Whole-Wheat Cinnamon Toast

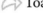

SUGAR AND SPICE AND EVERYTHING NICE COME WITH THIS LOVELY TREAT. THIS SNACK IS A GREAT SOURCE OF WHOLE GRAINS, AND RESEARCH SHOWS THAT CINNAMON MAY HELP TO LOWER LDL (BAD CHOLESTEROL) AND REGULATE OUR BLOOD SUGAR!

1 slice 100% whole-grain bread
1 tsp. butter
1 tsp. cinnamon
½ tsp. brown sugar

Toast bread and top with butter, cinnamon, and sugar.

YIELD: 1 serving
NUTRITION FACTS PER SERVING: 140 calories, 4.5g fat, 2.5g sat fat, 135mg sodium, 20g carbs, 3g fiber, 4g protein, 6% DV calcium, 8% DV iron.
TOTAL PREPARATION TIME: 3 minutes

Strawberry Milk Shake

THIS MILK SHAKE IS RICH IN NUTRIENTS, SUCH AS VITAMIN C, AND ANTIOXIDANTS, FOR WHICH STRAWBERRIES ARE KNOWN.

1 cup skim milk
¾ cup frozen strawberries
½ tbsp. honey

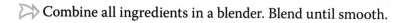 Combine all ingredients in a blender. Blend until smooth.

YIELD: 1 serving

NUTRITION FACTS PER SERVING: 160 calories, 0g fat, 0g sat fat, 130mg sodium, 30g carbs, 2g fiber, 10g protein, 10% DV vitamin A, 110% DV vitamin C, 25% DV calcium.

TOTAL PREPARATION TIME: 5 minutes

TREATS

Cubed Mangoes Dusted with Cinnamon

• • • • • •

MANGOES, WITH A LITTLE LESS THAN 3 GRAMS OF
FIBER PER CUP, ARE A VERY SATISFYING SNACK! TOP THIS
SWEET FRUIT WITH CINNAMON TO ADD A SAVORY,
SATISFYING FLAVOR!

1½ cups mangoes, cubed
2 tsp. cinnamon

➪ Sprinkle mango cubes with cinnamon and enjoy!

YIELD: 1 serving

NUTRITION FACTS PER SERVING: 160 calories, 1g fat, 0g sat fat, 0mg sodium, 41g
    carbs, 7g fiber, 2g protein, 50% DV vitamin A, 150% DV vitamin C, 8% DV
    calcium.

TOTAL PREPARATION TIME: 2 minutes

Berries and Whipped Cream Parfait

· · · · · ·

TAKE THIS CLASSIC BREAKFAST AND ADD SOME
WHIPPED CREAM TO MAKE THE PERFECT LIGHT
AFTER-DINNER TREAT!

¼ cup fat-free whipped topping
1 (6 oz.) container nonfat vanilla
    Greek yogurt
½ cup berries

⤳ Fold whipped topping into yogurt in a small bowl. Place half of
the yogurt mixture into a tall glass, top with berries and repeat for
2 more layers. Enjoy!

· ·

YIELD: 1 serving
NUTRITION FACTS PER SERVING: 160 calories, 0.5g fat, 0g sat fat, 95mg sodium, 32g
    carbs, 3g fiber, 6g protein, 15% DV vitamin A, 40% DV vitamin C, 20% DV
    calcium.
TOTAL PREPARATION TIME: 3 minutes

Hot Chocolate

• • • • • •

HAVE THIS HEALTHY WARM TREAT MADE FRESH,
WHICH IS AN EVEN BETTER OPTION THAN PREMIXED
PACKETS OF HOT CHOCOLATE, SINCE SOME VARIETIES
CONTAIN ARTIFICIAL SWEETENERS AND TRANS FATS.

1 cup skim milk
3 tbsp. cocoa powder
Pinch of stevia
1 tbsp. fat-free whipped topping

Warm the skim milk in a small saucepan over low heat. Stir in the cocoa powder and stevia until well combined. Top with whipped topping and enjoy!

YIELD: 1 serving
NUTRITION FACTS PER SERVING: 140 calories, 3g fat, 2g sat fat, 130mg sodium, 23g carbs, 3g fiber, 12g protein, 10% DV vitamin A, 25% DV calcium, 8% DV iron.
TOTAL PREPARATION TIME: 3 minutes

Strawberries and Dark Chocolate

• • • • • •

STRAWBERRIES ARE GREAT SOURCES OF VITAMIN C
AND MANGANESE! PAIR SWEET STRAWBERRIES WITH
SOME SAVORY CHOCOLATE. LOOK FOR DARK CHOCOLATE
WITH A COCOA CONTENT OF 70% OR MORE. QUALITY
DARK CHOCOLATE IN MODERATION MAY HELP REDUCE
HIGH BLOOD PRESSURE AND LDL (BAD CHOLESTEROL).

5 large strawberries, washed
1 oz. dark chocolate chips

⤳ Melt chocolate in the microwave for 30 seconds and stir until smooth. Dip strawberries into the chocolate and enjoy.

YIELD: 1 serving
NUTRITION FACTS PER SERVING: 160 calories, 9g fat, 5g sat fat, 0mg sodium, 21g carbs, 3g fiber, 2g protein, 50% DV vitamin C, 6% DV iron.
TOTAL PREPARATION TIME: 2 minutes

Parmesan Garlic Popcorn

· · · · · ·

POPCORN HAS MORE ANTIOXIDANTS THAN MOST
VEGETABLES! TAKE THIS GREAT SNACK, AND INSTEAD
OF PACKING ON THE CALORIES AND FAT WITH BUTTER,
SPRINKLE WITH PARMESAN AND GARLIC POWDER!

3 cups air-popped popcorn
½ tsp. extra-virgin olive oil
2½ tsp. shredded Parmesan
1 tsp. garlic powder

⇨ Drizzle olive oil over warm popcorn and toss with Parmesan and garlic powder to combine.

YIELD: 1 serving
NUTRITION FACTS PER SERVING: 150 calories, 5g fat, 1.5g sat fat, 75mg sodium, 21g carbs, 4g fiber, 6g protein, 6% DV calcium, 6% DV iron.
TOTAL PREPARATION TIME: 3 minutes

Banana Ice Cream

• • • • • •

BLEND FROZEN BANANAS, AND YOU ARE MAGICALLY
LEFT WITH ICE CREAM, WITHOUT THE SATURATED FAT
AND CALORIES!

1½ very ripe medium bananas,
   sliced

▷ Place bananas in a single layer on a baking sheet lined with parchment paper. Freeze for at least 2 hours. Then place frozen banana slices into a blender or food processor and blend until bananas reach the consistency of soft-serve ice cream!

YIELD: 1 serving
NUTRITION FACTS PER SERVING: 158 calories, 0.5g fat, 0g sat fat, 2mg sodium, 40g
   carbs, 4.5g fiber, 2g protein.
TOTAL PREPARATION TIME: 4 minutes plus 2 hours freeze time

Chocolate Avocado Pudding

• • • • • •

AVOCADOS ARE FULL OF HEALTHY FATS, WHICH
ADD A RICH, CREAMY TEXTURE TO THIS DECADENT
BUT GUILT-FREE PUDDING.

1 large ripe avocado, peeled and
chopped
½ cup skim milk
3 tbsp. liquid sweetener (like
honey or pure maple syrup)

3 tbsp. unsweetened cocoa
powder
½ tsp. vanilla extract

⤳ Place all ingredients in a blender and blend until very smooth.
Serve immediately or chill in the fridge and then enjoy.

YIELD: 3 servings
NUTRITION FACTS PER SERVING: 175 calories, 9.5g fat, 1.5g sat fat, 24mg sodium, 24g
carbs, 6g fiber, 3.5g protein, 9% DV vitamin C, 8% DV calcium, 8% DV iron.
TOTAL PREPARATION TIME: 5 minutes

PATTERN PORTIONS LIST

Vegetables

For all nonstarchy vegetables, the minimum serving size is 1 cup raw or ½ cup cooked, with the exception of salad greens, which have a minimum serving size of 2–3 cups raw. I say "minimum serving size" because you can't eat too many plain vegetables. If you add any fats in the cooking process (oils, butters, cheese, etc.) be sure to count them toward your allotted fat servings.

Fruits

One serving of fruit is one medium whole fruit or 1 cup chopped. Dried fruit has a serving size of 2 tbsp. Unsweetened applesauce and unsweetened canned fruit have a serving size of ½ cup.

Starches

Starches in the amounts listed below equal one starch serving (as indicated on your meal pattern). Choose starches that are whole grains or complex carbohydrates as often as possible.

Type	Food	Serving size
Bread	Bagel thin, 100% whole wheat	1
	Bread: pumpernickel, rye, unfrosted raisin, white, 100% whole grain or whole wheat	2 slices (80 calories or less per slice)
	100% whole-wheat sandwich thin	1
	Frozen waffles, 100% whole wheat	2 (170 calories or less per two waffles)
	English muffin, 100% whole wheat	1 (150 calories or less per muffin)
	Hamburger bun, 100% whole wheat	1 (150 calories or less per bun)
	Hot dog bun, 100% whole wheat	1 (150 calories or less per bun)
	Pancake (4 inches across, ¼ inch thick)	2
	Pita (6 inches across), 100% whole wheat	1 (150 calories or less per pita)
	Tortilla (6–8 inches across), corn or flour, 100% whole wheat	1 (150 calories or less per tortilla)
Cereals and grains	Barley, cooked	½ cup
	Bulgur wheat, cooked	½ cup
	Cereal: bran, whole-grain, spoon-size shredded wheat, frosted cereals	1 cup (less than 200 calories per cup)
	Oatmeal	½ cup
	Farro, cooked	½ cup
	Couscous, whole-grain	½ cup

	Granola, low-fat or regular	¼ cup
	Grits, cooked	½ cup
	Pasta, cooked, whole wheat	I cup
	Quinoa, cooked	½ cup
	Rice, cooked: white, brown	½ cup
	Tabbouleh, prepared	½ cup
	Wheat germ, dry	3 tablespoons
	Wild rice, cooked	½ cup
Starchy vegetables	Corn	½ cup
	Corn on the cob, large	½ cob (5 ounces)
	Mixed vegetables with corn, peas or pasta	I cup
	Parsnips	½ cup
	Peas or starchy beans	½ cup
	Potato, small to medium, baked with skin	I (5 ounces)
	Potato, mashed	½ cup
	Pumpkin, canned	I cup
	Squash: acorn, butternut	I cup
	Succotash	½ cup
	Yam or sweet potato, plain	½ cup or I small–medium whole (5 ounces)
Crackers and snacks	Popcorn, low-fat microwave or popped with no added fat	3 cups
	Rice cakes, whole-grain brown (4 inches across)	2
	Saltine crackers, whole-grain crackers (i.e., Triscuits)	6 (120 calories or less per 6 crackers)
	Snack chips, baked: tortilla, potato	I ounce (140 calories or less per I-ounce serving)

Dairy

Check the product label to see how much fat and how many calories each product contains. Stick to **fat-free or low-fat milk and yogurt products**, which contain 0 to 3 grams of fat and about 100 calories per serving. Low-fat dairy counts as a protein food for your meal pattern.

Type	Food	Serving size
Fat-free and low-fat milk and yogurt products	Low-fat (1% milk fat) buttermilk	1 cup (8 fluid ounces)
	Low-fat (1% milk fat) chocolate milk	1 cup (8 fluid ounces)
	Skim or low-fat (1% milk fat) milk	1 cup (8 fluid ounces)
	Yogurt, low-fat or fat-free, plain	6 ounces
	Yogurt, low-fat, fruit-flavored	6 ounces (130 calories or less per serving)
	Greek yogurt, low-fat or 0% fat, fruit-flavored	6 ounces (130 calories or less per serving)
	Greek yogurt, low-fat or 0% fat, plain	6 ounces
	Cottage cheese, low-fat	½ cup

Proteins

Choose **meatless and leanest animal proteins most often.** Proteins in the amounts listed below equal one serving.

Type	Food	Serving size
Meatless Proteins	*Note: Beans, peas, and lentils can be considered as either 1 lean protein serving or 1 starch serving. Count as a starch serving if having another protein serving in the same meal.*	
	Beans, cooked: black, garbanzo, kidney, lima, navy, pinto, white	½ cup

	Lentils, cooked: brown, green, yellow	½ cup
	Peas, cooked: black-eyed, split, green	½ cup
	Egg substitutes, plain	¼ cup
	Egg whites	2
	Whole eggs	1
	Veggie or bean burger	1 patty
	Tofu, all types	¾ cup (or 150 calories or less per serving)
Leanest Animal Protein	Beef, select or choice, trimmed of fat: 90% lean or leaner ground, roast, round, sirloin, tenderloin	4–5 ounces
	Fish, fresh or frozen: catfish, cod, flounder, haddock, halibut, orange roughy, salmon, tilapia, trout, tuna	4–6 ounces
	Hot dog	1 (3g fat or less per dog)
	Lamb: roast, chop, leg	4–5 ounces
	Luncheon meat: turkey, ham, chicken, roast beef	3–5 ounces (3g fat or less per ounce)
	Oysters, medium, fresh or frozen	6
	Pork, lean: Canadian bacon, chop, ham, tenderloin	4–5 ounces
	Poultry without skin: chicken, Cornish hen, duck, goose, turkey	4–5 ounces
	Sardines, canned	2 medium
	Shellfish: clams, crab, imitation shellfish, lobster, scallops, shrimp	4–6 ounces
	Tuna, canned in water or oil, drained	3–5 ounces
	Veal: loin chop, roast	4–5 ounces
	Wild game: buffalo, ostrich, rabbit, venison	4–5 ounces

Other Animal Proteins	Beef: corned beef, ground beef, meat loaf, prime rib, short ribs	3 ounces
	Fish, fried	3 ounces
	Lamb: ground, rib roast	3 ounces
	Pork: cutlet, shoulder roast	3 ounces
	Poultry: chicken with skin, fried chicken, ground chicken or turkey (skin, dark and light meat), duck	3 ounces
	Sausage	1 ounce (5g fat or less per ounce)
	Veal, cutlet, no breading	3 ounces

Fats

Fats in the amounts listed below equal one serving of fat. Remember to include any fats you use for cooking as part of your daily fat allowance. Choose monounsaturated and high polyunsaturated fats most often. *Note: Cheeses, nuts, or nut butters can count as a protein if no other source of protein is consumed at a meal.

Type	Food	Serving size
High monounsaturated fats	Avocado	2 tbsp. (or ¼ avocado)
	Olive, canola, or peanut oil	1 tsp.
	Black or green olives	8 large
	Nuts	2 tbsp. (may use ¼ cup if substituting for protein)
	Tahini paste	2 tsp.
	Seeds: sesame, sunflower, flax, pumpkin	1 tbsp.
	Nut butters (almond, peanut)	1 tbsp. (may use up to 2 tbsp. if substituting for protein)

High polyunsaturated fats	Light vegetable oil spread in a tub	1 tbsp.
	Trans-free stick or regular tub margarine	1 tsp.
	Mayonnaise, reduced-fat, canola, or olive oil mayo	1 tbsp.
	Mayonnaise, regular	1 tsp.
	Corn, soybean, safflower, or sunflower oil	1 tsp.
	Salad dressing, reduced fat	2 tbsp.
	Salad dressing, regular	1 tbsp.
	Reduced-fat/soft cheeses (goat)	1 oz. (or ¼ cup shredded or 2 tbsp. crumbled; may have up to 2 ounces if substituting for protein)
	Light cream cheese	2 tbsp.
High saturated fats	Whipped butter	2 tsp.
	Butter, reduced fat	1 tbsp.
	Butter stick	1 tsp.
	Bacon	1 slice
	Boiled chitterlings	2 tbsp.
	Half-and-half	2 tbsp.
	Cream cheese	1 tbsp.
	Hard cheeses (Parmesan, cheddar)	1 oz. (or ¼ cup shredded)
	Sour cream	1 tbsp.
	Palm, palm kernel, or coconut oil	1 tsp.
	Bacon grease	1 tsp.
	Coconut, sweetened or shredded	2 tbsp.
	Cream	1 tbsp.

MEAL PLANNING TOOL

Fill in the meal planner below at the beginning of each week to make staying on track a breeze!

MEAL PLANNER

Meal Pattern	Sunday	Monday	Tuesday
BREAKFAST			
1 serving starch			
1 serving protein			
1 serving fat			
1 serving fruit/veggies			
LUNCH			
1 serving starch			
1 serving protein			
1 serving fat			
2 servings fruit/veggies			
DINNER			
1 serving starch			
1 serving protein			
1 serving fat			
2 servings fruit/veggies			
SNACK			
1 serving fruit/veggie/starch			
1 serving protein/fat			
TREAT			
150 calories of whatever you want			

Wednesday	Thursday	Friday	Saturday

APPENDIX C

GROCERY LISTS AND PREP INSTRUCTIONS

Groceries

The grocery lists below correspond to the two-week menu plan in Chapter 4. If you would like to have the Plan B meal ingredients on hand, be sure to check out the Plan B grocery list below so you can shop for those items once per month.

Also, be aware that some recipes make multiple servings, while other recipes make only one serving. This variety adds the flexibility for you to choose recipes that work best for you. For example, if you are preparing meals for your family, you may want to choose the recipes that make multiple servings. The grocery lists have the right amount of ingredients to make the number of servings listed in each recipe's yield, and many of the recipes with higher yields are used for leftover-based lunches in your menu plan. If you wish to make more or less of any dish, be sure to take a look at the recipes and adjust your grocery list accordingly.

The grocery lists below assume that you have some staples, such as the spices and herbs mentioned in Chapter 6, salt and pepper, cooking spray, brown sugar/stevia, flour, butter, extra-virgin olive/canola oils, honey, vanilla extract, cocoa powder, lower-sodium chicken broth, citrus (lemon/lime) juice, garlic, balsamic vinegar, peanut butter, light vinaigrette salad dressing, and basic condiments.

GROCERY LIST WEEK 1

GRAINS AND BREAD

- 1-lb. box quinoa
- 1 loaf 100% whole-wheat bread
- 1 box (at least 4 single-serving packets) instant unflavored oatmeal
- 1 package (at least 10) 8-inch whole-wheat tortillas (with about 80 calories per tortilla, such as La Tortilla Factory)
- small package whole-grain granola (you will need about ½ cup)

DAIRY AND EGGS

- 6 large eggs
- 1½ cup shredded part-skim mozzarella cheese
- 16 oz. nonfat plain Greek yogurt
- 8 oz. low-fat cottage cheese
- 8 oz. crumbled Feta cheese

PRODUCE

- 6 medium bananas
- 4½ cups baby carrots
- 16 cups fresh baby spinach
- 4 medium apples
- 1 cup blueberries
- 2 large tomatoes
- 2 large portabella mushroom caps

- ➤ 2 cups (16 oz.) sliced white mushrooms
- ➤ 1 medium yellow onion (or 1 cup presliced onion from your produce department)
- ➤ 1 medium head Bibb lettuce
- ➤ 1 medium baking potato
- ➤ 1 large container strawberries (about 4 cups)
- ➤ 1 large bell pepper
- ➤ 1 large bunch grapes from California (about 3 cups)
- ➤ 1 medium cucumber

NUTS, SEEDS, DRIED FRUITS, AND OTHER
- ➤ 1 small box raisins
- ➤ 1 medium package dry-roasted almonds (you will need about 2 cups)
- ➤ 1 small package seasoned sun-dried tomatoes (such as Bella Sun Luci with Greek oregano, basil, and garlic)
- ➤ 1 medium bag sliced almonds (you will need about 1 cup)
- ➤ 2 oz. dark-chocolate-covered almonds
- ➤ 1 package popcorn kernels (you will need enough to make 6 cups popped)
- ➤ 1 small bag dark chocolate chips (you will need less than 1 cup)

DELI AND BAKERY
- ➤ 20 oz. fresh salsa
- ➤ 6 oz. roast beef deli meat (have the deli slice just this amount for you)
- ➤ 2 hard-boiled eggs
- ➤ 12 oz. hummus

CANNED/BOTTLED/SPECIAL SAUCES OR SEASONINGS
- ➤ 5 (3 oz.) cans salmon
- ➤ 1 (5 oz.) can chunk light tuna in water
- ➤ 1 (15½ oz.) can chickpeas

- 1 (15½ oz.) can black beans
- ground flaxseed
- blackened seasoning
- Old Bay seasoning
- 1 large jar marinara sauce (about 2 cups)
- cocoa powder

FROZEN
- 1 small bag (single-serving) seasoned mixed vegetables
- 1 package whole-grain waffles, such as Van's

MEAT/FISH
- 4 (4 oz.) salmon fillets, skin removed

GROCERY LIST WEEK 2

DAIRY AND EGGS
- 1 half gallon skim milk
- 1 (24 oz.) container plain nonfat Greek yogurt
- 2 (6 oz.) containers vanilla nonfat Greek yogurt
- 16 oz. soft goat cheese
- 2 cups shredded cheese of your choice

PRODUCE
- 1 large container strawberries (about 4 cups)
- 4 medium bananas
- 2 large portabella mushroom caps
- 1 large avocado
- 3 cups spinach
- 3 cups baby carrots
- 1 lemon
- 2 cups blueberries
- 1 medium apple

- 4 large tomatoes
- 4 medium zucchini
- 1½ cups chopped white or yellow onion (look for prechopped packages in your produce department)
- 2 large bell peppers
- 1 large bunch basil (optional)
- 2 small baking potatoes
- 3 cups chopped fresh kale
- 1 large mango (or look for 1½ cups presliced mango in your produce department)
- 4 large sweet potatoes (enough to make 7 cups when chopped—or look for 7 cups prechopped sweet potatoes in your produce department)

DELI AND BAKERY
- 1 whole-grain baguette

CANNED/BOTTLED/SPECIAL SAUCES OR SEASONINGS
- 1 (15½ oz.) can black beans
- 1 (5 oz.) can chunk light tuna packed in water
- 1 (15½ oz. or smaller) can lentils

FROZEN
- 1 small container fat-free whipped topping (you will need less than 1 cup)
- 4 cups frozen mixed vegetables + 1 small bag (single-serving) steam-in-microwave mixed vegetables
- 4 (6 oz.) tilapia fillets

MEAT/FISH
- 1 lb. lean ground beef (at least 90% lean or leaner)
- 8 (4 oz.) boneless, skinless chicken breasts that can be cooked from frozen

YOU SHOULD ALSO HAVE THESE ITEMS LEFT OVER FROM WEEK 1

- ½ pound dry quinoa
- 3 packets of instant unflavored oatmeal
- dark chocolate chips
- fresh salsa
- 3 eggs
- 5 slices 100% whole-wheat bread
- 4 100% whole-wheat tortillas
- seasoned sun-dried tomatoes
- hummus
- marinara
- sliced almonds
- dry-roasted almonds
- popcorn kernels
- dark chocolate almonds
- whole-grain frozen waffles
- ¼ cup granola
- raisins

PLAN B MEALS GROCERY LIST

The items on this list will allow you to have all ingredients on hand to make all six Plan B meals. This grocery list also assumes you have the staples mentioned at the beginning of this appendix. Plan B meals do not require any additional prep at the beginning of the week. Items denoted by an asterisk (*) should be stored in the fridge or freezer to extend their shelf life.

GRAINS AND BREAD

- microwavable quinoa or you can substitute brown rice if you can't find microwavable quinoa (at least 4 cooked cups' worth)
- 1 (16 oz.) box whole-wheat pasta

➤ 1 small package 100% whole-wheat sandwich thins*
  ➤ 1 small package corn tortillas*
  ➤ 1 standard-size large bag baked tortilla chips (140 calories per ounce)

DAIRY AND EGGS

➤ Parmesan cheese* (check label to see if it requires refrigeration)

PRODUCE

➤ 1 large sweet potato

NUTS, SEEDS, AND DRIED FRUIT

➤ 1 small package pine nuts*
➤ 1 small package seasoned sun-dried tomatoes, such as Bella Sun Luci with Greek oregano, basil and garlic* (check label to see if it requires refrigeration after opening)

CANNED/BOTTLED

➤ small jar salsa*, after opening
➤ 1 (5 oz.) canned chunk light tuna packed in water
➤ 1 (15½ oz.) can chickpeas
➤ 1 (6 oz.) can diced chicken breast
➤ 1 (3 oz.) can diced chicken breast
➤ 4 (15 oz.) cans pineapple tidbits in 100% juice
➤ 2 (15½ oz.) cans lower-sodium chicken broth
➤ 3 (15 oz.) cans black beans
➤ 3 (14½ oz.) cans whole kernel corn
➤ 1 (14½ oz.) can crushed tomatoes

FROZEN

➤ 1 box veggie burger patties (such as MorningStar Farms' Chipotle Black Bean)*
➤ 1 small bag shelled edamame*

> diced red onion (at least 2½ cups)*
  > diced yellow onion (at least 1 cup)*
  > chopped spinach (at least 2¼ cups)*
  > 4 (5 oz.) fillets frozen salmon that can be cooked from frozen (such as Gorton's Classic Grilled Salmon)*
  > Mixed vegetables (at least 10 cups)*

OILS, SPICES, HERBS, AND SEASONINGS
> Mrs. Dash Southwest Chipotle seasoning
> smoked paprika

Prep for Week 1

After you come home from the grocery store with your Week 1 meal plan supplies, take a few minutes to do the following prep work. This will make your meals during the week come together in a flash!

1. Wash and chop 8 baby carrots and ¼ cup spinach. Store together in a plastic baggie for your **On-the-Go Omelet.**
2. Wash and chop/slice:
   > *¾ cup spinach*
   > *4 medium apples. Toss in lemon or lime juice to prevent browning.*
   > *2 tomatoes*
   > *2 onions if you were unable to find the prechopped package version*
   > *1 cup strawberries*
   > *1 large bell pepper*
   > *8 baby carrots*
   > *1 medium cucumber*
3. Cook half the package of the quinoa according to package directions.

4. Prepare the salmon and chickpea mixture for the **Salmon and Chickpea Lettuce Wraps** according to the recipe.
5. Freeze 1¼ cups grapes and 1½ peeled and sliced bananas in separate freezer-safe baggies for treats.

Prep for Week 2

1. Wash and chop/slice:
   - *⅔ + ½ cup strawberries*
   - *¾ cup spinach*
   - *1 medium apple. Toss in lemon or lime juice to prevent browning.*
   - *7 cups sweet potatoes*
   - *8 baby carrots*
   - *4 cups zucchini*
   - *1 large mango (if you could not find presliced in your produce department)*
2. Cook all the quinoa according to package directions.
3. Freeze 1½ bananas in freezer-safe baggies for Banana Ice Cream and freeze ¾ cup chopped Strawberries for Strawberry Milk Shake.

ACKNOWLEDGMENTS

Writing my first book has been a wonderful experience, and there are many people who have helped me along the way. First, I would like to thank my husband for his patience throughout this process and for sharing my love of food and cooking. Also, I would like to thank our families for their constant love and support.

A special thank-you goes out to my agent, Hannah Gordon of Foundry Literary + Media, as well as to my editor, Jennifer Schuster, and the whole team at New American Library and Penguin for being wonderful to work with and holding my hand through this entire process.

Thank you to my brother-in-law, Adam Bedwell, PT, DPT, for reviewing the exercises suggested in this book.

A big thank-you to intern Alexis Joseph for her help with the research, recipes, and much more, as well as to interns Mairead Callahan and Kyle Smithson for their help with recipe testing and analysis. Thank you to my talented photographer, Ron Manville, for making my recipes come to life through images and for encouraging me along the way.

Thank you to all the amazing registered dietitians in my life who encourage me, give me advice, and inspire me!

Disclosures: I am a spokesperson or consultant to the following brands/products mentioned in this book: National Cattlemen's Beef Association, CLIF Bar and Company (Luna), California Table Grape Commission, National Mango Board, and Welch's.

SCHEDULE ME SKINNY
REFERENCES

CHAPTER 1

1. People who eat 34 grams of fiber per day absorb 6% fewer calories.
   - *Baer, David J., et al. Dietary fiber decreases the metabolizable energy content and nutrient digestibility of mixed diets fed to humans.* Journal of Nutrition *127, no. 4 (1997): 579–86.*

CHAPTER 2

1. Information on carbohydrates, proteins, and fats
   - *http://www.nutrition411.com/*
2. This is because research shows that when we consume carbohydrates, particularly whole-grain carbohydrates, they stimulate our brains to release serotonin, a hormone that helps us feel relaxed and satisfied after a meal.
   - *Salomon, Sharon. Boost mood with whole foods: Ban*

processed foods in lieu of nutrient-rich, whole foods, such as fruits, vegetables, fish, and whole grains to elevate your mood. Environmental Nutrition *(2012).*

> ➤ *Schaechter, J., and R. Wurtman. Serotonin release varies with brain tryptophan levels. Brain Research 532 (1990): 203–10.*
> ➤ *Wurtman, R. Nonnutritional uses of nutrients.* European Journal of Pharmacology *668 (2011): S10–S15.*

3. Studies also show that people who eat whole grains have less belly fat than those who don't. I don't know about you, but that sounds like a good excuse to me to eat a nice, comforting serving of whole-grain pasta. Take that, you depriving low-carb diets!

> ➤ *McKeown, N., L. Troy, P. Jacques, U. Hoffmann, C. O'Donnell, and F. Fox. Whole and refined-grain intakes are differentially associated with abdominal visceral and subcutaneous adiposity in healthy adults: The Framingham Heart Study.* American Journal of Clinical Nutrition *92 (2010): 1165–71.*

4. Bean eaters weigh less and have slimmer stomachs.

> ➤ *http://wwwn.cdc.gov/nchs/nhanes/bibliography/key_statistics.aspx*

5. People who ate eggs for breakfast lost 65% more weight.

> ➤ *Vander Wal, J. S., A. Gupta, P. Khosla, and N. V. Dhurandha. Egg breakfast enhances weight loss.* International Journal of Obesity *32 (2008): 1545–55.*

6. Resistant starch may promote burning and shrinking of fat cells.

> ➤ *Slavin, Joanne L. Carbohydrates, dietary fiber, and resistant starch in white vegetables: Links to health outcomes.* Advances in Nutrition *4 (2013): 3515–55.*

7. Women who eat oily fish have lowest levels body fat.

> ➤ *Jackobsen, M. U., et al. Fish consumption and subsequent change in body weight in European women and men.* British Journal of Nutrition *109, no. 2 (2013): 353–62.*

CHAPTER 3

1. Let's start with breakfast. One of the number one nutrition mistakes that people make is eating little or no breakfast. This can cause your metabolism to slow down and make you feel low on energy. In fact, a study from Virginia Commonwealth University in Richmond found that obese women who ate a 600-calorie breakfast shed about 40 pounds in eight months, but those who ate a low-calorie breakfast experienced weight loss of only about 9 pounds.

    ➤ *Jakubowicz, D.,* The Big Breakfast Diet *(2009).*

2. Dieters who ate a sweet with their breakfast lost 40 pounds more (and kept it off) than those who ate low-calorie, low-carb breakfasts.

    ➤ *Jakubowicz, D., O. Froy, J. Wainstein, and M. Boaz. Meal timing and composition influence ghrelin levels, appetite scores, and weight loss maintenance in overweight and obese adults.* Steroids *77 (2012): 323–31.*

3. Brown-bagging it is the easiest way to keep things balanced at lunch. You have probably already heard that bringing your lunch can be better for both your health and your wallet. In fact, you can save almost $3,000 per year if you switch to bringing your lunch instead of buying it. But you and your lunch-box-toting kids may be getting tired of the same old, same old sandwich-and-fruit routine.

    ➤ *http://moneylicious.org/infographic-brown-bagging-packing-a-lunch-could-save-you-3000-a-year/*

4. Studies show that mindful eaters eat less without even trying and feel more satisfied with the food they do eat.

    ➤ *Wansink, B.* Mindless Eating: Why We Eat More Than We Think. *New York, NY: Bantam, 2007, 1–112.*

5. A recent study from the *Journal of the American Dietetic Association* found that dieters who noshed between breakfast

and lunch tended to snack later in the day, too. And the calories added up. Morning snackers lost 4% less weight in a year than did those who skipped the midmorning snack.

> *Kong, A., et al. Associations between snacking and weight loss and nutrient intake amount postmenopausal overweight to obese women in a dietary weight-loss intervention.* Journal of the American Dietetic Association *111 (2011): 1898–1903.*

CHAPTER 4

1. Scientists at the University of Tennessee found that people on a reduced-calorie diet who included an extra 300 to 400 mg of calcium a day lost significantly more weight than those who ate the same number of calories but with less calcium. Scientists aren't exactly sure why, but eating calcium-rich foods is more effective than taking calcium supplements.

> *Zemel, Michael B. Role of calcium and dairy products in energy partitioning and weight management.* American Journal of Clinical Nutrition *79, no. 5 (2004): 907S–912S.*

2. Antioxidants

> *Crujeiras, Ana B., et al. A role for fruit content in energy-restricted diets in improving antioxidant status in obese women during weight loss.* Nutrition *22, no. 6 (2006): 593–99.*

> *Ello-Martin, Julia A., et al. Dietary energy density in the treatment of obesity: A year-long trial comparing two weight-loss diets.* American Journal of Clinical Nutrition *85, no. 6 (2007): 1465–77.*

> *Masaki, H. Role of antioxidants in the skin: Anti-aging effects.* Journal of Dermatological Science *58, no. 2 (2010): 85–90.*

➤ Mozaffarieh, M., S. Sacu, and A. Wedrich. *The role of the carotenoids, lutein and zeaxanthin, in protecting against age-related macular degeneration: A review based on controversial evidence.* Nutrition Journal 20, no. 2 (2001): 1–8.

➤ Perrig, W. J., P. Perrig, and H. B. Stahelin. *The relation between antioxidants and memory performance in the old and very old.* Journal of the American Geriatric Society 45, no. 6 (1997): 718–24.

➤ Rao, A. V., and S. Agarwal. *Role of antioxidant lycopene in cancer and heart disease.* Journal of the American College of Nutrition 19, no. 5 (2000): 563–69.

➤ Kline, K., K. Lawson, W. Yu, and B. Sanders. *Vitamin E and cancer.* Vitamins and Hormones 76 (2007): 435–61.

➤ Park, H. J., et al. *Vitamin C attenuates ERK signaling to inhibit the regulation of collagen production by LL-37 in human dermal fibroblasts.* Experimental Dermatology 19, no. 8 (2010): e258–e264.

➤ Massaro, M., et al. *Omega-3 fatty acids, inflammation, and angiogenesis: Basic mechanisms behind the cardioprotective effects of fish and fish oils.* Cellular and Molecular Biology 56, no. 1 (2010): 59–82.

➤ Kiecolt-Glaser, J. K., et al. *Omega-3 supplementation lowers inflammation and anxiety in medical students: A randomized controlled trial.* Brain, Behavior, and Immunity 25, no. 8 (2011): 1725–34.

➤ Jicha, G. A., and W. R. Markesbery. *Omega-3 fatty acids: Potential role in the management of early Alzheimer's disease.* Clinical Interventions in Aging 5 (2010): 45–61.

➤ Cassidy, A., et al. *High anthocyanin intake is associated with a reduced risk of myocardial infarction in young and middle-aged women.* Circulation 127 (2013): 188–96.

➤ De Amicis, F., et al. *Resveratrol, through NF-Y/p53/Sin3/ HDAC1 complex phosphorylation, inhibits estrogen receptor gene expression via p38MAPK/CK2 signaling in human breast cancer cells.* FASEB Journal 25, no. 10 (2011): 3695– 3707.

➤ Seidman, M. D., et al. *Resveratrol decreases noise-induced cyclooxygenase-2 expression in the rat cochlea.* Otolaryngology Head and Neck Surgery 148 (2013): 827–33.

➤ Qin, F., et al. *The polyphenols resveratrol and S17834 prevent the structural and functional sequelae of diet- induced metabolic heart disease in mice.* Circulation 125 (2012): 1757–64.

➤ Goldberg, L. J., and Y. Lenzy. *Nutrition and hair.* Clinics in Dermatology 24, no. 4 (2010): 412–19.

➤ Pandey, K. B., and S. B. Rizvi. *Plant polyphenols as dietary antioxidants in human health and disease.* Oxidative Medicine and Cellular Longevity 2, no. 5 (2009): 270–78.

➤ Mukhtar, H. *Eat plenty of green leafy vegetables for photoprotection emerging evidence.* Journal of Investigative Dermatology 121, no. 2 (2003): viii.

➤ Rosenblum, Jennifer L., et al. *Calcium and vitamin D supplementation is associated with decreased abdominal visceral adipose tissue in overweight and obese adults.* American Journal of Clinical Nutrition 95, no. 1 (2012): 101–8.

➤ Johnston, Carol S. *Strategies for healthy weight loss: From vitamin C to the glycemic response.* Journal of the American College of Nutrition 24, no. 3 (2005): 158–65.

➤ Zittermann, Armin, et al. *Vitamin D supplementation enhances the beneficial effects of weight loss on cardiovascular disease risk markers.* American Journal of Clinical Nutrition 89, no. 5 (2009): 1321–27.

> *Major, Geneviève C., et al. Supplementation with calcium + vitamin D enhances the beneficial effect of weight loss on plasma lipid and lipoprotein concentrations.* American Journal of Clinical Nutrition 85, no. 1 (2007): 54–59.

> *Parra, Dolores, et al. A diet rich in long chain omega-3 fatty acids modulates satiety in overweight and obese volunteers during weight loss.* Appetite 51, no. 3 (2008): 676.

> *Mori, Trevor A., et al. Dietary fish as a major component of a weight-loss diet: Effect on serum lipids, glucose, and insulin metabolism in overweight hypertensive subjects.* American Journal of Clinical Nutrition 70, no. 5 (1999): 817–25.

CHAPTER 5

1. According to the Food Marketing Institute, for every minute we spend in the grocery store, we spend $2!
   > *http://www.clemson.edu/extension/hgic/food/nutrition/food_shop_prep/food_shop/hgic4221.html*
   > *Brookshire Grocery's bakeries hit all customer levels. Modern Baking, May 23, 2011.*
   > *Couldn't find the exact URL of the food marketing institute. The statistic is referenced in both of these publications*

2. Next, look, but don't touch. If an item is not on your list—even if it looks interesting—do not pick it up. If you pick up an item, you are four times more likely to buy it than if you don't touch it.
   > *http://www.craftsreport.com/show-business/30-how-to-get-customers-4x-more-likely-to-buy.html*

3. A recent study found that people who use a basket are three times more likely to pick up junk food than people who use a cart!

> *Van den Bergh, B., J. Schmitt, and L. Warlop. Embodied myopia.* Journal of Marketing Research *48, no. 6 (2011): 1033–44.*

4. Store brands (or generics) tend to be the same quality as name-brand food items, and the store brands have a price tag that is already 20% cheaper.

> *http://www.eatright.org/Public/content. aspx?id=5493&terms=coupons*

5. Meat and Poultry Tips: When possible and affordable, opt for . . .

> *Meat and Poultry Labeling Terms. USDA Food Safety and Inspection Service. United States Department of Agriculture, 12 Apr. 2011. Web. 29 May 2013. http://www.fsis.usda.gov/ factsheets/meat_&_poultry_labeling_terms/.*

> *Daley, Cynthia A., et al. A review of fatty acid profiles and antioxidant content in grass-fed and grain-fed beef.* Nutrition Journal *9, no. 1 (2010): 10.*

> *DellaValle, C. T., et al. Dietary intake of nitrate and nitrite and risk of renal cell carcinoma in the NIH-AARP Diet and Health Study.* British Journal of Cancer *108, no. 1 (2012): 205–12.*

> *Easton, M. D. L., D. Luszniak, and E. Von der Geest. Preliminary examination of contaminant loadings in farmed salmon, wild salmon and commercial salmon feed.* Chemosphere *46, no. 7 (2002): 1053–74.*

> *Hamilton, M. Coreen, et al. Lipid composition and contaminants in farmed and wild salmon.* Environmental Science and Technology *39, no. 22 (2005): 8622–29.*

> *Knekt, Paul, et al. Risk of colorectal and other gastro-intestinal cancers after exposure to nitrate, nitrite, and N-nitroso compounds: A follow-up study.* International Journal of Cancer *80, no. 6 (1999): 852–56.*

> Kant, Ashima K., Barry I. Graubard, and Arthur Schatzkin. *Dietary patterns predict mortality in a national cohort: The National Health Interview Surveys, 1987 and 1992.* Journal of Nutrition *134, no. 7 (2004): 1793–99.*

CHAPTER 6

1. Pepperine reduces activity of genes that form fat cells.

   > *http://pubchem.ncbi.nlm.nih.gov/summary/summary. cgi?cid=638024*

CHAPTER 7

1. Next time you go out to eat, notice if the colors red or yellow are used anywhere on the menu. Studies show that these colors tend to stimulate the appetite. Often, certain "special" items may be printed in red while simple items remain printed in black and white. It's easy for your eyes to skip over these items and be drawn to the bright colors. So read your menu carefully to avoid missing a good choice.

   > Singh, S., *Impact of color on marketing.* Management Decision *44, no. 6 (2006): 783–89.*

2. Also, to keep us paying more, restaurants often add extra charges to get something prepared a certain way or to split an entrée. Many times their hope is that we will be turned off by this charge and end up ordering two separate entrées. But since studies show we eat most of what's on our plates, we are likely to both eat and pay more overall than had we just paid the $5 to split the plate.

   > Ittersum, K. V., and B. Wansink. *Plate size and color suggestibility: The Delboeuf illusion's bias on serving and*

eating behavior. Journal of Consumer Research *39, no. 2 (2012): 215–28.*

CHAPTER 8

ENERGY BOOSTING NUTRIENTS

1. **B Vitamins:** The B vitamins, found in foods like eggs, leafy greens, whole grains, and legumes, play a critical role in energy metabolism. B-complex vitamins fuel the brain by helping to metabolize carbohydrates, so a deficiency can lead to serious fatigue. Eating a varied diet full of fruits, vegetables, whole grains, and lean meats is a surefire way to ensure adequate intake of the B vitamin complex.

   - *Heap, L. C., T. J. Peters, and S. Wessely. Vitamin B status in patients with chronic fatigue syndrome.* Journal of the Royal Society of Medicine *92, no. 4 (1999): 183.*

   - *Werbach, Melvyn R. Nutritional strategies for treating chronic fatigue syndrome.* Alternative Medicine Review *5, no. 2 (2000): 93–108.*

2. **Zinc:** If you're feeling fatigued, especially during exercise, make sure your zinc levels are adequate. Zinc is essential for all of the enzymes involved in energy metabolism, so low zinc levels can leave you feeling sluggish. You can find it in foods such as milk, meat, chicken, beans, and nuts. It's critical for healthy hair, skin, bones, and overall physical growth.

   - *Cordova, A., and M. Alvarez-Mon. Behaviour of zinc in physical exercise: A special reference to immunity and fatigue.* Neuroscience and Biobehavioral Reviews *19, no. 3 (1995): 439–45.*

3. **Omega-3 Fatty Acids:** Research shows a strong correlation between depression and low levels of omega-3 fatty acids. Because chronic fatigue syndrome is a common comorbidity of major depression, it's important to get plenty of omega-3 fatty

acids to boost energy and fight fatigue. Get your dose by consuming fatty fish like sardines, mackerel, salmon, and tuna, as well as plant sources like flaxseed.

> *Maes, M., I. Mihaylova, and J.-C. Leunis. In chronic fatigue syndrome, the decreased levels of omega-3 poly-unsaturated fatty acids are related to lowered serum zinc and defects in T cell activation.* Neuroendocrinology Letters 26, no. 6 (2005): 745–51.

4. **Vitamin C:** Vitamin C is a potent immune-boosting anti-oxidant, but it also plays a key role in enhancing energy when it comes to physical performance. Citrus fruits like kiwis, oranges, and strawberries or veggies like bell peppers are chock-full of this stuff, so get chomping to minimize muscle weakness and fatigue. Quick tip: Vitamin C also helps aid in the absorption of iron!

> *Lukaski, H. C. Vitamin and mineral status: Effects on physical performance.* Nutrition 20, nos. 7–8 (2004): 632–44.

5. Potassium helps your body to convert the calories from food you eat into energy that your body can use.

> *Panel on Dietary Reference Intakes for Electrolytes and Water, Standing Committee on the Scientific Evaluation of Dietary Reference Intakes. Dietary Reference Intakes for Water, Potassium, Sodium, Chloride, and Sulfate. Washington, DC: National Academies Press, 2004.*

6. Magnesium plays a role in metabolism, nerve function, and muscle function. When magnesium levels are low, the body produces more lactic acid, the same substance that is produced after a hard workout, which induces fatigue.

> *Volpe, Stella Lucia. Magnesium in disease prevention and overall health.* Advances in Nutrition: An International Review Journal 4, no. 3 (2013): 378S–383S.

> *Panel on Dietary Reference Intakes for Calcium, Phosphorus, Magnesium, Vitamin D, and Fluoride, Standing Committee*

on the Scientific Evaluation of Dietary Reference Intakes.
Dietary Reference Intakes for Water, Potassium, Sodium,
Chloride, and Sulfate. Washington, DC: National
Academies Press, 2004.

WATER

1. Even slight dehydration can cause a decrease in energy.

- Armstrong, L. E., et al. Mild dehydration affects mood in
  healthy young women. Journal of Nutrition 142, no. 2 (2012):
  382–88.
- Kraft, J. A., et al. Impact of dehydration on a full body
  resistance exercise protocol. European Journal of Applied
  Physiology 109, no. 2 (2010): 259–67.
- Campbell, S. M. Hydration needs throughout the lifespan.
  Journal of the American College of Nutrition 26, suppl. 5
  (2007): 585S–587S.
- Shaw, G. How much water should you drink when you exercise?
  WebMD. N.p., n.d. Web. June 11, 2013. http://www.webmd.
  com/fitness-exercise/features/water-for-exercise-fitness.
- Latzka, William A., and Scott J. Montain. Water and
  electrolyte requirements for exercise. Clinics in Sports
  Medicine 18, no. 3 (1999): 513–24.
- Valtin, Heinz. "Drink at least eight glasses of water a day."
  Really? Is there scientific evidence for "8×8"? American
  Journal of Physiology—Regulatory, Integrative, and
  Comparative Physiology 283, no. 5 (2002): R993–R1004.

SLEEP

1. Harvard scientists found that people who sleep for fewer than
   5 hours per night are much more likely to gain weight over the
   course of a year than people who sleep a full 7 hours.

- Patel, S. R., et al. Association between reduced sleep and *weight gain in women.* American Journal of Epidemiology *164 (2006): 947–54.*

EXERCISE

1. In fact, studies show that three 10-minute exercise sessions are just as effective as one 30-minute session.

    ➤ *Schmidt, W. D., C. J. Biwer, and L. K. Kalscheuer. Effects of long versus short bout exercise on fitness and weight loss in overweight females.* Journal of the American College of Nutrition *20, no. 5 (2001): 494–501.*

    ➤ *Hazell, T. J., et al. Two minutes of sprint-interval exercise elicits 24-hour oxygen consumption similar to that of 30 minutes of continuous endurance exercise.* International Journal of Sport Nutrition and Exercise Metabolism *22, no. 4 (2012): 276–83.*

COFFEE AND CAFFEINE

➤ *Cassel, Daisha. Benefits of java: Health benefits of drinking coffee.* Academy of Nutrition and Dietetics, *April 2013. Web. 29 May 2013.*

➤ *Evans, Suzette M., and Roland R. Griffiths. Caffeine tolerance and choice in humans.* Psychopharmacology *108, nos. 1–2 (1992): 51–59.*

➤ *Huxley, Rachel, et al. Coffee, decaffeinated coffee, and tea consumption in relation to incident type 2 diabetes mellitus: A systematic review with meta-analysis.* Archives of Internal Medicine *169, no. 22 (2009): 2053.*

➤ *Mesas, Arthur Eumann, et al. The effect of coffee on blood pressure and cardiovascular disease in hypertensive individuals: A systematic review and meta-analysis.* American Journal of Clinical Nutrition *94, no. 4 (2011): 1113–26.*

➤ *"Should I give up caffeine now that I am pregnant?"*
Nutrition Q & A. Academy of Nutrition and Dietetics, n.d.
Web. 29 May 2013.

➤ *"The Buzz on Caffeine." Tip of the Day. Academy of*
Nutrition and Dietetics, n.d. Web. 29 May 2013.

➤ *Higdon, Jane V., and Balz Frei. Coffee and health: A review*
of recent human research. Critical Reviews in Food Science
and Nutrition *46, no. 2 (2006): 101–23.*

➤ *Lopez-Garcia, Esther, et al. Changes in caffeine intake and*
long-term weight change in men and women. American
Journal of Clinical Nutrition *83, no. 3 (2006): 674–80.*

➤ *Westerterp-Plantenga, Margriet S., Manuela PGM Lejeune,*
and Eva MR Kovacs. Body weight loss and weight
maintenance in relation to habitual caffeine intake and
green tea supplementation. Obesity Research *13, no. 7*
(2005): 1195–1204.

➤ *Bell, Douglas G., and Tom M. McLellan. Exercise endurance*
1, 3, and 6 h after caffeine ingestion in caffeine users and
nonusers. Journal of Applied Physiology *93, no. 4 (2002):*
1227–34.

➤ *"Medicines in My Home: Caffeine and Your Body." U.S. Food*
and Drug Administration, Apr. 2007. Web. 6 June 2013.

➤ *http://www.fda.gov/downloads/Drugs/ResourcesForYou/*
Consumers/BuyingUsingMedicineSafely/
UnderstandingOver-the-CounterMedicines/UCM205286.
pdf.

➤ *"Nutrition by the Cup." Beverage Nutrition Information.*
Starbucks Coffee Company, 2011. Web. 6 June 2013. http://
globalassets.staStarbucks.ca/menu/nutrition.

➤ *"The Buzz on Energy-Drink Caffeine." Energy Drinks.*
Consumer Reports, *December 2012. Web. 6 June 2013.*

➤ *http://www.consumerreports.org/cro/magazine/2012/12/*
the-buzz-on-energy-drink-caffeine/index.htm.

CHAPTER 9

1. That's because mindful eaters tend to eat less and still feel more satisfied.
   - ➤ *Beshara, Monica, Amanda D. Hutchinson, and Carlene Wilson. Does mindfulness matter? Everyday mindfulness, mindful eating, and self-reported serving size of energy dense foods among a sample of South Australian adults.* Appetite *(2013).*
   - ➤ *Kidd, Lori I., Christine Heifner Graor, and Carolyn J. Murrock. A mindful eating group intervention for obese women: A mixed methods feasibility study.* Archives of Psychiatric Nursing *(2013).*

2. Studies show that people eat more when they are standing up than when they are sitting down.
   - ➤ *Remick, Abigail K., Janet Polivy, and Patricia Pliner. Internal and external moderators of the effect of variety on food intake.* Psychological Bulletin *135, no. 3 (2009): 434–51.*

3. That's because the size of dinner plates has increased by about 23% in just the past 20 years!
   - ➤ *Young, Lisa R., and Marion Nestle. The contribution of expanding portion sizes to the US obesity epidemic.* American Journal of Public Health *92, no. 2 (2002): 246–49.*

4. Cornell researchers found that just by switching from a 12-inch plate to a 10-inch plate, you could consume up to 22% fewer calories!
   - ➤ *Wansink, Brian. From mindless eating to mindlessly eating better.* Physiology and Behavior *100, no. 5 (2010): 454–63.*
   - ➤ *Wansink, Brian. Environmental factors that unknowingly increase a consumer's food intake and consumption volume.* Annual Review of Nutrition *24 (2004): 455–79.*

5. A study from the *Journal of Consumer Research* found that

people served themselves a larger portion of food when its color was close to the color of the plate.

> ➤ *Van Ittersum, Koert, and Brian Wansink. Plate size and color suggestibility: The Delboeuf illusion's bias on serving and eating behavior.* Journal of Consumer Research *39, no. 2 (2012): 215–28.*

6. That's because research has proven time and time again that people eat more when they are not solely focused on the food.

> ➤ *Hetherington, Marion M., et al. Situational effects on meal intake: A comparison of eating alone and eating with others. Physiology and Behavior 88, no. 4 (2006): 498–505.*

7. A study from the *American Journal of Clinical Nutrition* reported that people who ate in front of the TV consumed more food and were more likely to describe their meal as unsatisfying as well.

> ➤ *Robinson, Eric, et al. Eating attentively: A systematic review and meta-analysis of the effect of food intake memory and awareness on eating.* American Journal of Clinical Nutrition *97, no. 4 (2013): 728–42.*

> ➤ *Temple, Jennifer L., et al. Television watching increases motivated responding for food and energy intake in children.* American Journal of Clinical Nutrition *85, no. 2 (2007): 355–61.*

CHAPTER 10

1. Studies show that the more variety of foods we have to choose from, the more we'll eat.

> ➤ *Foote, Janet A., et al. Dietary variety increases the probability of nutrient adequacy among adults.* Journal of Nutrition *134, no. 7 (2004): 1779–85.*

2. People who keep a food journal lose twice as much weight as those who don't.

> ➤ *Hollis, Jack F., et al., Weight loss maintenance trial research group, weight loss during the intensive intervention phase of the weight-loss maintenance trial.* American Journal of Preventive Medicine *35, no. 2 (2008): 118–26.*

INDEX